DIAGNOSTIC PROBLEMS IN TUMOR PATHOLOGY SERIES

DIAGNOSTIC PROBLEMS IN TUMORS OF FEMALE GENITAL TRACT: SELECTED TOPICS

DIAGNOSTIC PROBLEMS IN TUMOR PATHOLOGY SERIES

Series Editors

Arun Chitale, MD (Path)

Diplomate American Board of Pathology (1969)

Surgical Pathologist Sir HN Hospital, Jaslok Hospital,

Surgical Pathology Center

Formerly Professor & Head Department of Pathology Bombay Hospital Institute of Medical Sciences, Mumbai, India

Dhananjay Chitale, MD (Path) DNB,

Diplomate American Board of Pathology

Division Head, Molecular Pathology & Genomic Medicine,

Senior Staff Surgical Pathologist

Director, Tissue Biorepostiroy

Assistant Clinical Professor, Wayne State University School of Medicine

Henry Ford Hospital, Detroit, Michigan, USA

Diagnostic Problems in Tumors of Head and Neck: Selected Topics, 1/e
Arun Chitale, Dhananjay Chitale, 2014
Diagnostic Problems in Tumors of Gastrointestinal Tract: Selected Topics, 1/e
Arun Chitale, Dhananjay Chitale, 2014
Diagnostic Problems in Tumors of Female genital Tract: Selected Topics, 1/e
Arun Chitale, Dhananjay Chitale, 2014

Published by Arun Chitale & Dhananjay Chitale

Copyright © 2014 Chitale publications

DIAGNOSTIC PROBLEMS IN TUMOR PATHOLOGY SERIES

DIAGNOSTIC PROBLEMS IN TUMORS OF FEMALE GENITAL TRACT: SELECTED TOPICS

Authors

Kedar Deodhar, MD (Path), MRCpath
Professor & Pathologist
Tata Memorial Hospital, Mumbai, India

Arun Chitale, MD (Path)
Diplomate American Board of Pathology (1969)
Surgical Pathologist
Sir HN Hospital, Jaslok Hospital, Surgical Pathology Center
Formerly Professor & Head Department of Pathology Bombay Hospital Institute of Medical Sciences, Mumbai, India

Table of Contents

PREFACE:	VII
DISCLAIMER:	VIII
Tumors of the uterine corpus	1
Endometrial tumors	2
Endometrioid Adenocarcinoma of Endometrium & variants	2
Cellular classification of Endometrial Carcinoma	2
Endometrial Hyperplasia	3
WHO Classification of Endometrial hyperplasia [1]	3
Endometrioid Adenocarcinoma with Squamous Differentiation	7
Serous adenocarcinoma of endometrium	9
Serous Endometrial Cancers (SC) That Mimic Endometrioid Carcinomas (EC)	10
Endometrial Intraepithelial Carcinoma (EIC)	12
Serous carcinoma arising in endometrial polyp	12
Clear Cell Carcinoma of Endometrium (CCC)	13
Endometrial Adenocarcinoma in Women under 40 years of Age	15
Malignant Mixed Mullerian Tumors (MMMT)	16
Mullerian Adenosarcoma (MA)	23
Endometrial Stromal Tumor (EST)	25
Current Classification of ESS	25
Low Grade Endometrial Stroma Sarcoma	25
Endometrial Stromal Nodule	30
Uterine smooth muscle tumors	32
Leiomyosarcoma (LMS)	32
Smooth Muscle Tumor of Uncertain Malignant Potential (STUMP)	32
Atypical leiomyoma	34
Epithelioid Smooth Muscle Tumors	36
Tumors of the uterine cervix	38
Minimal Deviation Adenocarcinoma of Cervix	39
Glandular Lesions of Cervix Mimicking Adenocarcinoma	42
Deep cervical glands and cysts:	42
Tuboendometrioid Metaplasia (TEM) and Endometriosis	42
Microglandular Adenosis (MGA) or hyperplasia	43
Mesonephric remnants	46
Endocervical Glandular Dysplasia	47
Malignant Melanoma of Female Genital Tract	50
Mucosal Melanoma	50
Vulvar Melanoma	50
Paget's disease of Vulva	51
Vaginal Melanoma	52
Cervical Melanoma	53
Sarcoma Botryoides (Embryonal Rhabdomyosarcoma)	54
Gestational Trophoblastic diseases	56
WHO Classification of Gestational Trophoblastic diseases	56
Placental site trophoblastic tumor (PSTT)	56
Exaggerated placental site reaction(synonymous with "Syncitial endometritis")	59
Placental Site Nodule/Plaque (PSN-P)	59

- Tumors of the Ovary 60
  - Surface Epithelial Tumors 61
  - Serous borderline tumors (SBT) Synonyms: 61
  - Serous borderline tumors with microinvasion 63
  - 'SBT with micropapillary pattern' or is it micropapillary carcinoma? 65
  - Serous borderline tumors with lymph node involvement 66
  - Serous Carcinomas of Ovary 67
  - Mucinous borderline tumors 68
  - Mucinous Borderline Tumors 69
  - MBT of intestinal type 69
  - Intraepithelial carcinoma and microinvasion in intestinal MBT 70
  - MBT: ovarian primary or metastatic mucinous carcinoma 70
  - Pseudomyxoma Peritonei (PMP) 71
  - Clear cell carcinoma of the ovary 75
  - Gonadoblastoma (Germ cell-sex cord-stromal tumor) 77
  - Metastatic Tumors in ovaries ("Krukenberg tumors") 80
  - Distinction between Primary and Metastatic Mucinous Carcinomas of the Ovary 80
  - Aggressive Angiomyxoma (AAM) 84
  - PEComa of the Female Genital Tract 87
  - Fallopian Tube Serous Carcinoma &Molecular Pathogenesis of Ovarian Carcinoma 89
  - References 91

PREFACE:

DIAGNOSTIC PROBLEMS IN TUMOR PATHOLOGY:

Uncommon presentation of common lesions and rare lesions

Histopathological evaluation is the gold standard in the diagnosis of malignant tumors and chronic diseases of visceral organs like liver, kidney and lungs. Histopathological analysis provides information that helps the clinician to choose the most appropriate treatment modality and assists in prognostication. Notwithstanding the current and future advances in the imaging technology and other innovations, the status of Histopathology will remain unchanged for decades to come.

Whereas Histopathology is the most objective form of investigation, there are many gray areas in arriving at a definitive diagnosis. On many occasions total lack of clinical information leads to avoidable errors in the diagnosis. The surgical pathologist is advised to keep the cases pending until adequate information is available. On the other hand there are numerous problems in histological interpretation even if the entire clinical information is at hand. This occurs because some lesions have inherent morphological ambiguities and no two surgical pathologists may agree on the correct histological diagnosis. One such lesion, for example, is verrucous squamous cell carcinoma of the oro-pharyngeal region or other organs with squamous epithelial lining. The most controversial problem in thyroid disorders is a lesion called follicular variant of papillary carcinoma. In every organ and system, there are sporadic entities, which have debatable criteria of morphological diagnosis. The object of this book is to adequately address problems of uncommon morphologic variations of common lesions and rare difficult lesions with the help of extensive illustrations. There are excellent frequently updated textbooks of surgical pathology, in which all lesions occurring in various sites are described, illustrated and backed by references. However, due to constraints of space, these problematic entities are not extensively illustrated or explained at length. This deficiency is admirably handled in exclusively individual organ pathology monograms. However, this requires the facility of a well-stocked library; most practicing surgical pathologists do not have access to these.

The proposed book is an attempt to address these lesions with multiple illustrations and detailed pertinent text. It is envisaged that the book should be a companion to a standard surgical pathology textbook and this should be accessible just at the fingertips via power of electronic media using internet. The targeted audience includes residents in Anatomic Pathology; young recently qualified pathologists and a large contingent of pathologists attached to medical institutions, in which the volume of surgical specimens is low.

Note on statistical data presented in this eBook:

The senior author (ARC) has been a practicing consultant surgical pathologist for the last 44 years (1969-2013). As a surgical pathologist, he has been associated with 'surgical pathology center' (his own lab). He is also attached to the following hospitals in Mumbai (Bombay): Sir H N Hospital, Bombay Hospital and Jaslok Hospital (all corporate institutions), Bone Registry, Grant Medical College; Cytology department of KEM Hospital.

He has gathered vast amount of neoplastic cases of different organ-systems and the data has been in the form of Tables for different organ systems. The statistical tabulation of tumors has been based on classification of anatomical site and behavior (benign or malignant). This is not purported to be a population based epidemiological data. However, the data likely represents a fair cross sectional distribution and representation of various neoplasms in the population served in Metropolitan Mumbai (Bombay), India.

DISCLAIMER:

This Book titled Diagnostic Problems in Tumors of Female Genital Tract: Selected Topics, is made available by the Authors solely for trained and licensed physician for personal, non-commercial teaching and educational use. No two individual patients with neoplasms are identical and therefore diagnosis and treatment varies greatly depending on the medical and surgical history. The information contained in this Book is not medical advice. It is the professional responsibility of the practitioner to apply the information provided in a specific situation. Attention has been taken for accuracy of the information presented to describe generally accepted practices; however, knowledge and best practice in the field constantly change with new research. Readers are advised to check the most current information. The authors, editors and publishers are not responsible for errors or omissions or for any outcomes from the use of the information in this book and make no warranty, expressed or implied, with respect to the currency, completeness or accuracy of the content of the publication. This educational application is not a medical device and does not and should not be construed to provide health related or medical advice, or clinical decision support or to support or replace the diagnosis, recommendation, advise, treatment or decision by an appropriately trained licensed physician, including, without limitation with respect to any life sustaining or lifesaving treatment or decision. This educational material does not create a physician patient relationship between the authors and any individual. Before making any medical or health related decision, individuals, including those with any neoplasms are advised to consult an appropriately trained and licensed physician. To the fullest extent of the law, the authors, the editors or the publisher do not assume any liability for any injury and/or damage to persons or property arising out of or related to any use of the material contained in this book.

ENDOMITERIAL TUMORS

Tumors of the uterine corpus

Table 1:Tumors of uterine corpus (n = 9521) Authors series (1970-2006) Epithelial Tumors (*n* = 982)	
Endometrioid Adenocarcinoma (Grade III: 15 %)	858 (87.37%)
Adenoacanthoma	68 {6.90%)
Adenosquamous carcinoma	31 (3.15%)
Clear Cell Carcinoma	10 (1.01%)
Serous Carcinoma**	08 (0.96%)
Transitional cell Carcinoma	02 (0.24%)
Squamous Cell Carcinoma (Without cervical involvement)	05 (0.51%)

Benign Mesenchymal Tumors of Uterus (*n* = 8268)	
Leiomyoma	8059 (97.4%)
Epithelioid Leiomyoblastoma	7 (.08%)
Adenomyoma	200 (2.4%)
Lipoma	02 (0.024%)
Adenomyosis: 3365 cases – an entity not included in tumors)	

Malignant Mesenchymal Tumors of Uterus (n = 142)	
Leiomyosarcoma	23 (16.2%)
Malignant Mixed Mullerian Tumor	40 (28.16%)
Mullerian Adenosarcoma	6 (4.2%)
Endolymphatic Stromal Myosis ***	3 (2.1%)
Endometrial Stromal Nodule	12 (8.5%)
Endometrial Stromal Sarcoma	58 (40.8%)

** the proportion of serous carcinomas of endometrium in the table above is significantly lower than reported in the literature because in the past, serous adenocarcinomas were labeled as high grade endometrial adenocarcinoma

*** Endometrial stromal myosis has a unique histological pattern and cases are separately listed, but these are all low grade endometrial stromal sarcomas

Endometrial tumors

Endometrioid Adenocarcinoma of Endometrium & variants

Worldwide, endometrial carcinoma is the fifth most common cancer in women. It is the third most common cause of gynecologic cancer deaths (behind ovarian and cervical cancer). About 3 decades back, endometrial carcinoma was labeled endometrial adenocarcinoma regardless of degree of anaplasia or any apparent deviant pattern. Over the years, many subtypes have been recognized. Bokhman JV in 1983 1, described two pathogenetic types of endometrial carcinomas, Type I and Type II.

In the past two decades, clinicopathologic, immunohistochemical, and molecular genetic studies have provided data to allow for the development of a dualistic model of endometrial carcinogenesis.

Type I

Type I endometrial carcinoma represents an estrogen-related tumor, which usually arises in the setting of endometrial hyperplasia, has low grade endometrioid histology, tends to be biologically indolent and accounts for 80% to 85% of cases. The term endometrioid is derived from the fact that the neoplastic glands resemble the glands of normal proliferative phase endometrium. A few morphological variants of this carcinoma are listed below and there is no prognostic difference among the subtypes. Unopposed estrogenic stimulation is the driving force behind this group of tumors. It may be the result of anovulatory cycles that occur in young women with the polycystic ovary syndrome. Patients with Type I endometrial cancers are frequently obese, diabetic, nulliparous, hypertensive or have late menopause.

Type II

The type II cancers are not estrogen-derived; display a high grade morphology, tendency for deep myometrial infiltration, and a poor prognosis. Serous carcinoma and clear cell carcinoma are the prototype of this group of endometrial carcinomas and will be discussed in detail.

Cellular classification of Endometrial Carcinoma

I) Endometrioid [account for 75% to 80%]
   (A) Ciliated
   (B) Secretory
   (C) Papillary or Villoglandular
   (D) Adenocarcinoma with squamous differentiation
II) Uterine papillary serous (10%)
III) Clear cell
IV) Mucinous
V) Squamous cell
VI) Transitional cell
VII) Small cell
VIII) Mixed
IX) Undifferentiated

Endometrial Hyperplasia

Endometrial hyperplasia (EH) is a precursor lesion of type I endometrial adenocarcinoma and there is some confusion about the correct histological interpretation and nature of this lesion in terms of malignant transformation.

Definition

EH represents a non-physiological, non-invasive proliferation of the endometrium that results in morphological pattern of glands with irregular shapes, varying sizes, and increase in gland-stroma ratio.

WHO Classification of Endometrial hyperplasia [1]

Simple hyperplasia without atypia
Simple hyperplasia with atypia

Complex (adenomatous) hyperplasia without atypia
Complex (adenomatous) hyperplasia with atypia

Clinical Features

Hyperplasia is frequently found in the endometrial curettings, which is carried out for investigation of infertility. It is due to anovulation, which also accounts for abnormal bleeding occurring in peri-menopausal women. Postmenopausal women developing hyperplasia are usually on unopposed estrogen hormone replacement therapy and manifest abnormal bleeding. It is of interest and instruction to know that atrophy is the most common cause of uterine bleeding in postmenopausal women. In one study of 226 cases of women with postmenopausal bleeding, 56% had atrophy, 15% had various types of hyperplasia and only 7% showed carcinoma[2].

Microscopic

Simple Hyperplasia previously referred to as cystic glandular hyperplasia, shows proliferating glands of irregular size and shape and with focal cystic appearance. The glands are unevenly crowded and separated by abundant endometrial stroma. Cytologically, the glandular epithelium resembles proliferative type endometrium (Figure 1 A-C).

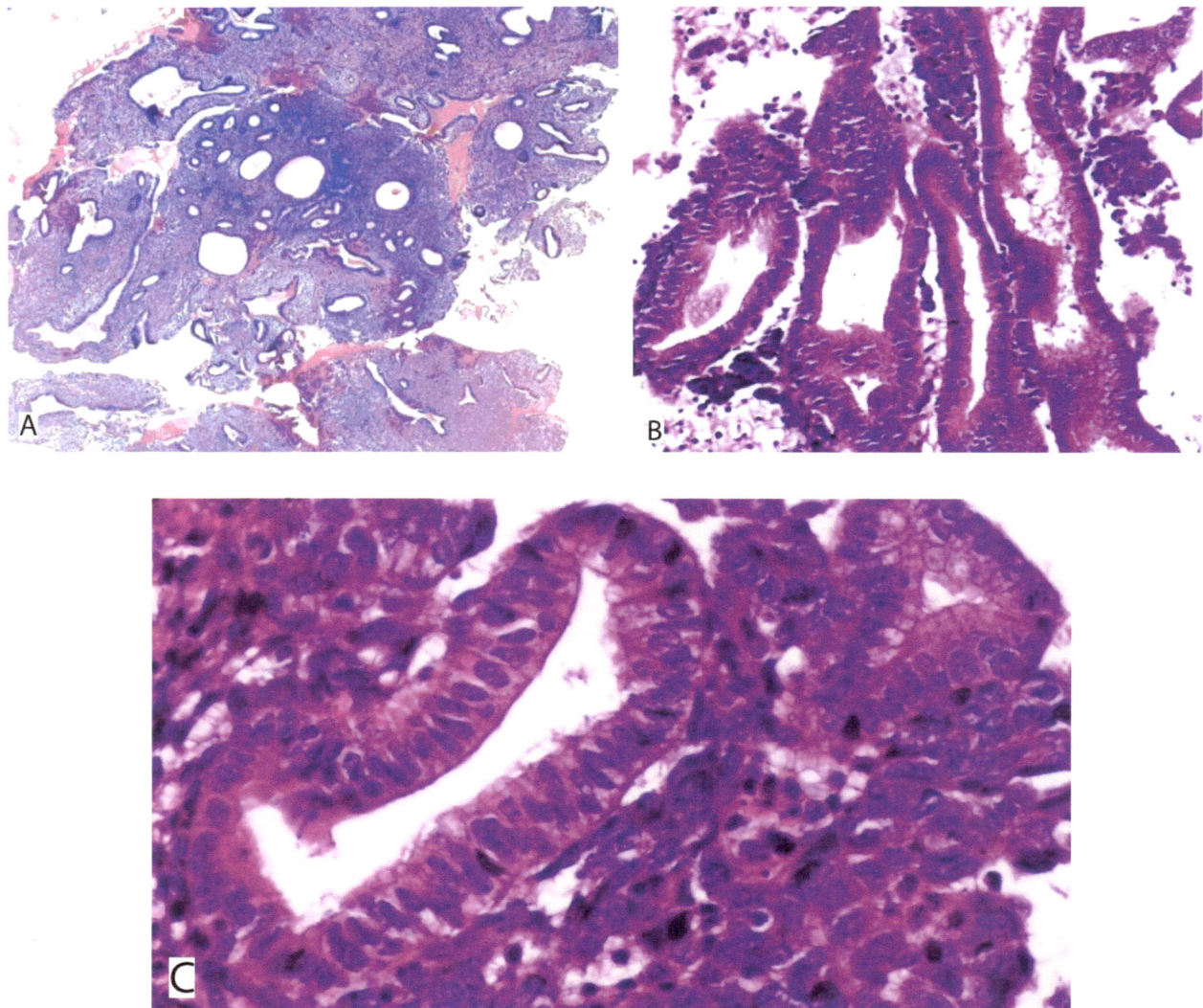

Figure 1(A) Scanner view of simple hyperplasia with cystic glands; (B and C) thick hyperplastic crowded enlarged endometrial glands, with minimal stroma and without atypia

Complex Hyperplasia, previously termed adenomatous hyperplasia, shows more densely crowded glands, which display structural complexity with more outpouchings and infoldings. The glands are typically closely packed and represent a back-to-back pattern with minimal intervening endometrial stroma. There should be at least twice as many glands as stroma in any field for gland-stroma ratio of more than 2:1 3.

Simple Atypical Hyperplasia as an entity may fit into the WHO classification of hyperplasia but it has been observed that most cases of atypical hyperplasia have a complex pattern with closely apposed glands (complex atypical hyperplasia). In a large retrospective analysis, no case of simple atypical hyperplasia has been found in retrospective screened material. In similar publications, it is assumed that this category, if it does exist, is extremely rare. 4, 5, 6

In case of Complex Atypical Hyperplasia (Figure 2 A-D), the glands are highly irregular in size and shape, sometimes associated with papillary infoldings projecting in the lumen. The single most important feature to distinguish between non-atypical and atypical hyperplasia is the presence of nuclear atypia. The cytological atypia is represented by loss of axial polarity, often with rounding of nuclei, high N/C ratio, irregular nuclear membranes, nuclear clearing and nucleoli. Atypia is nearly always focal in distribution. Figure 2 (E, F) reveals overlap of complex atypical hyperplasia with well-differentiated adenocarcinoma. In the long term follow up studies fewer than 2% hyperplasia without cytological atypia progressed to carcinoma, whereas 23% of hyperplasia with cytological atypia progressed to carcinoma. 7, 8, 9

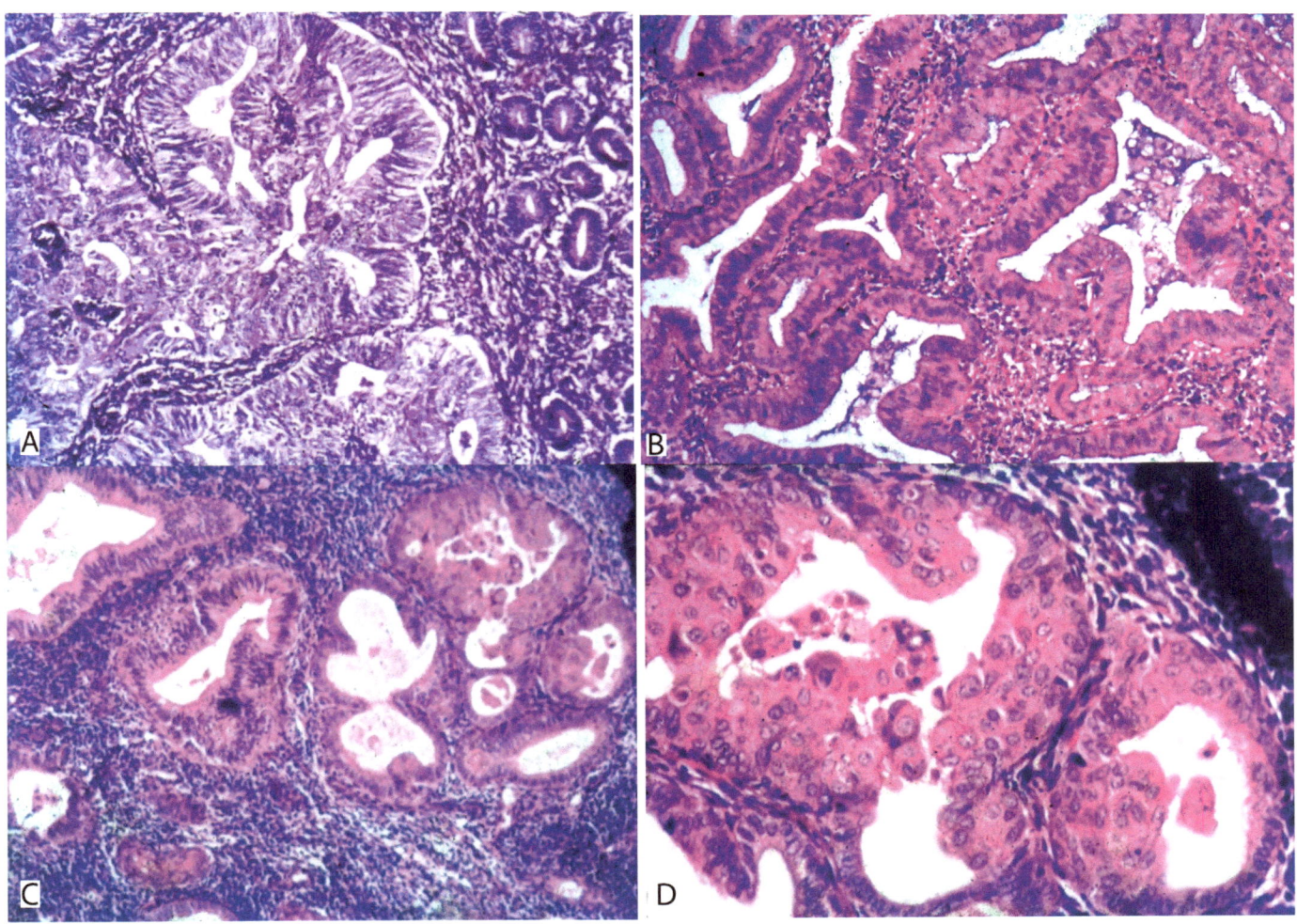

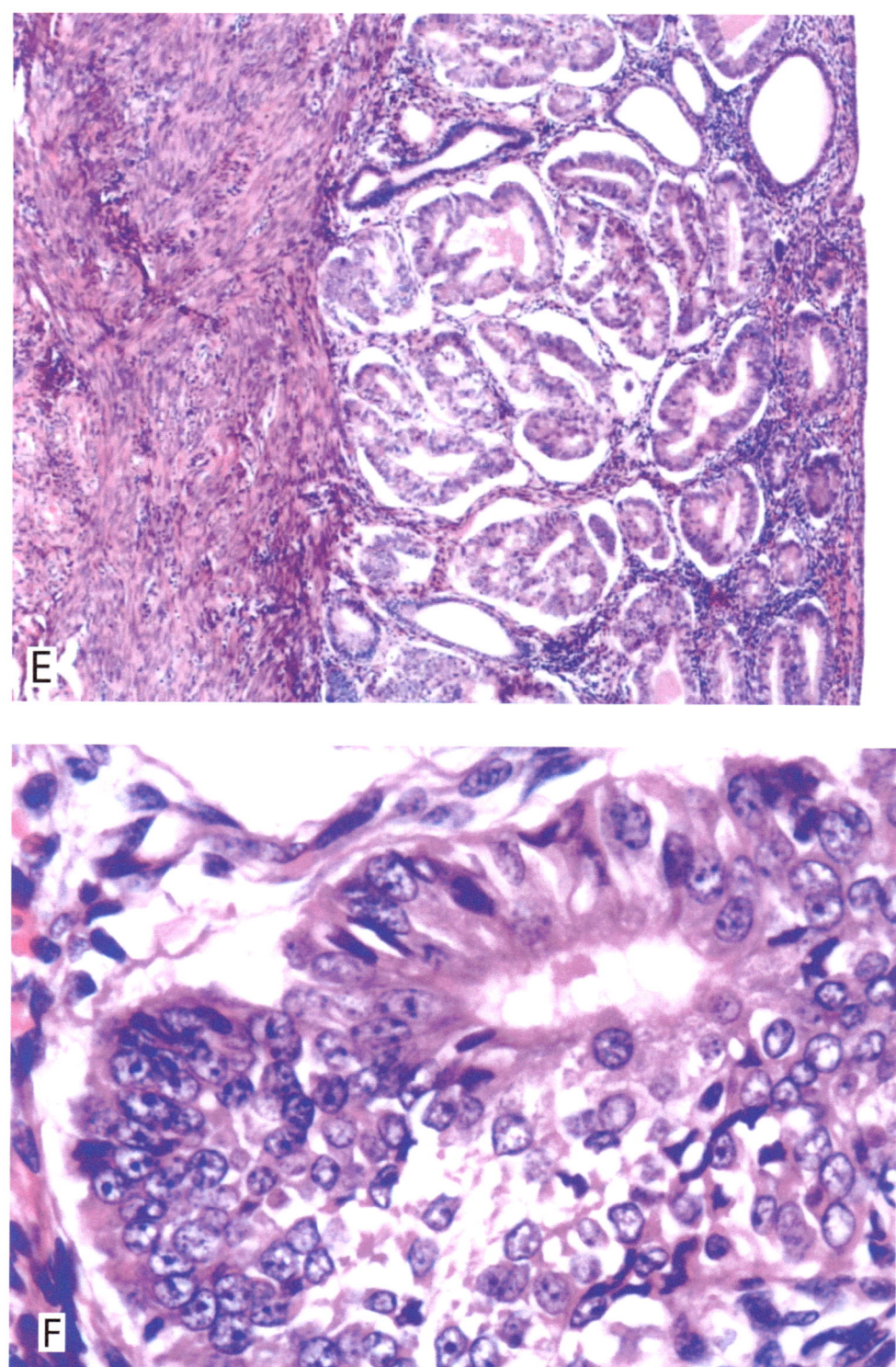

Figure2 (A-D) Various histological appearances of complex atypical hyperplasia of endometrium (E) low power view of Complex Atypical Hyperplasia with suspicion of well differentiated adenocarcinoma, Situated beneath a thin atrophic endometrial mucosa with no myometrial invasion; (F) close up view shows enlarged stratified nuclei

Endometrioid Adenocarcinoma with Squamous Differentiation

Squamous differentiation is identified in about 25% cases of endometrial adenocarcinoma. However, its biological significance has been a subject of debate for decades. The squamous component may appear benign, malignant or indeterminate and in majority of instances closely follows the differentiation of the glandular component. The benign component manifests in the form of groups of mature (keratinised) epithelial cells or solid nests of oval or short spindle cells (squamous morules) emanating from endometrial glands. If foci of squamous metaplasia are prominent or extensive, the tumor is designated as Adenoacanthoma (AA) (Figure 3 A-B), a term that has been in use since about 1911 10.

In the 1970s, examples of endometrial adenocarcinoma having cytological features of malignancy in the squamous component have been reported in the literature. This tumor has been, since then, identified as adenosquamous carcinoma (AS) (Figure 3 C-D). WHO definition for adenosquamous carcinoma (AS): a tumor in which adenocarcinomatous and squamous carcinomatous elements are intermingled. A survey of 675 cases of endometrial cancer seen in a 20-year period showed that the incidence of adenosquamous carcinoma was 5%. The authors reported that prognosis of adenosquamous carcinoma was worse than that for pure endometrial adenocarcinoma 11.

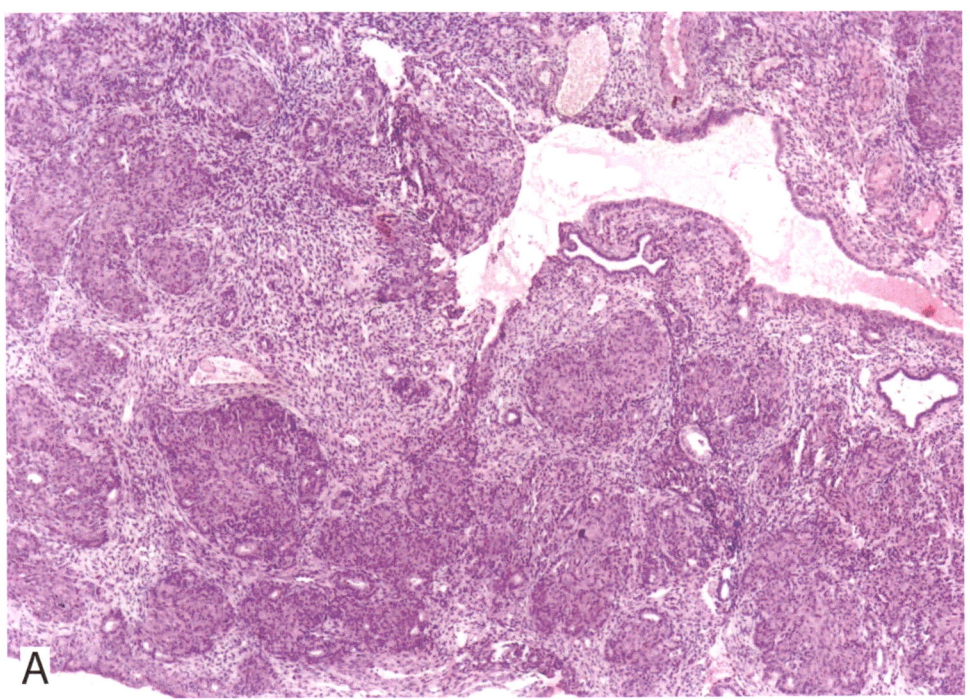

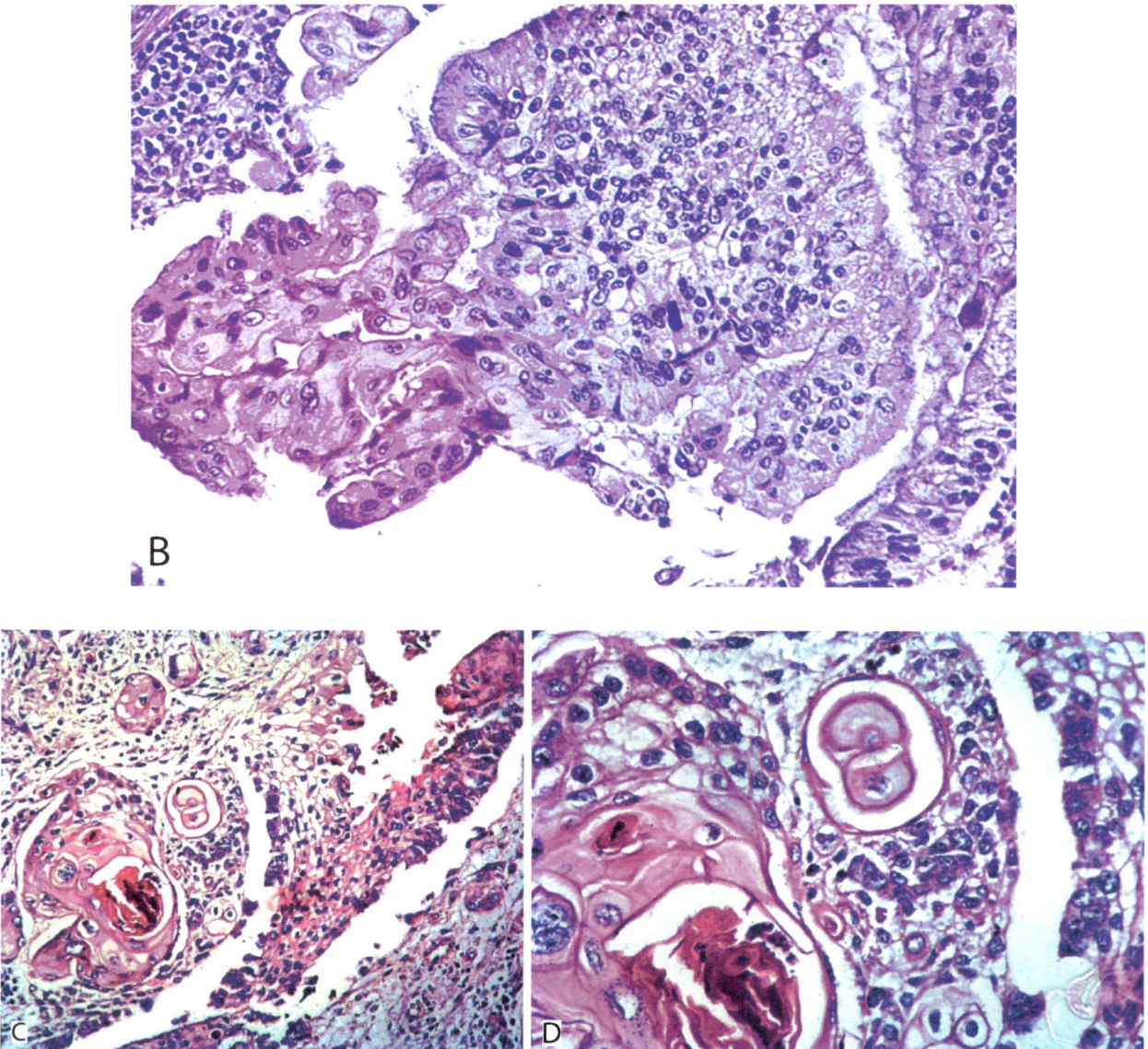

Figure 3 (A, B) Adenoacanthoma (endometrioid adenocarcinoma with squamous differentiation); (C, D) Adenosquamous carcinoma of endometrium

Many have advocated that AA and AS terms be replaced by the descriptive term adenocarcinoma with squamous differentiation. We do not believe that this is necessary because there is no confusion in the nomenclature: AA stands for adenocarcinoma with squamous metaplasia and AS for adenocarcinoma with squamous carcinoma. This is reproducible because squamous metaplasia can be easily differentiated from anaplasia of squamous cell carcinoma. The only issue is whether adenosquamous carcinoma has poorer prognosis than pure adenocarcinoma. The data of Norwegian Cancer Registry has shown that pure endometrial adenocarcinoma has better prognosis than adenosquamous carcinoma 12.

Prognosis

The report of Norwegian Cancer Registry 12 on 1985 cases of endometrial adenocarcinoma revealed 181 cases (9.1%) of Adenoacanthoma and 74 cases (3.7%) of adenosquamous carcinoma. The survival rates were as follows:

91.2% and 79.6% five-year and ten-year survival rates for Adenoacanthoma
64.9% and 52.7% five-year and ten-year survival rates for Adenosquamous carcinoma

This data from Norwegian Cancer Registry confirms the existence of adenosquamous carcinoma as an entity and that its prognosis is poorer than that of adenoacanthoma. It has been noted that survival rate for Adenoacanthoma is similar to or slightly better than that for endometrioid adenocarcinoma. The incidence of myometrial invasion and survival Figures of AS are similar to those of poorly differentiated endometrial adenocarcinoma. Myometrial invasion is a very important factor, regardless of grade, in the long-term prognosis. It is recommended that Pathologists should provide information on histological grade, depth of myometrial invasion and presence of vascular involvement or spread to the cervix in all cases of endometrial carcinoma to help the clinician formulate appropriate treatment 13.

Serous adenocarcinoma of endometrium

Definition

Endometrial papillary serous carcinoma (SC) is a histological subtype of endometrial adenocarcinoma that is characterized by papillary architecture, high grade nuclear anaplasia and advanced stage at initial presentation 14. It behaves more aggressively than endometrioid adenocarcinoma.

Clinical Findings

The prevalence of SC reported from various referral centers is usually about 10% and prevalence rate is 1% in a population based study from Norway 15. In our own experience, only 8 cases of SC were detected among 982 endometrial adenocarcinomas (1%, Table I). This is mainly due to delay in our recognition of existence of endometrial serous carcinoma (SC). It is highly likely that some cases of (SC) have been reported as poorly differentiated endometrioid adenocarcinoma in the past. Women with SC are older (mean ages in late sixties), typically postmenopausal in contrast to women with endometrioid carcinoma. Cases of SC usually give no history of estrogen therapy and are more likely to have abnormal cervical cytology.

Gross

Uteri containing these tumors are usually atrophic and the growth generally exophytic. It is difficult to assess the presence of myometrial invasion on gross examination alone. In some cases, an endometrial polyp is associated with growth, and the polyp has been thought to be a precursor lesion for SC.

Microscopic

Although a papillary pattern predominates, glandular or solid patterns also occur. A fibro vascular framework identical to that encountered in ovarian serous carcinoma supports the papillary pattern. The stroma supporting the papillae is often edematous or broad and provides stromal network on which are arranged highly pleomorphic and hyperchromatic epithelial cells. The cells of SC may possess prominent nucleoli 16. The cells are cuboidal or typically hobnail shaped and the cytoplasm acidophilic or vacuolated (Figure 4 A-D)).

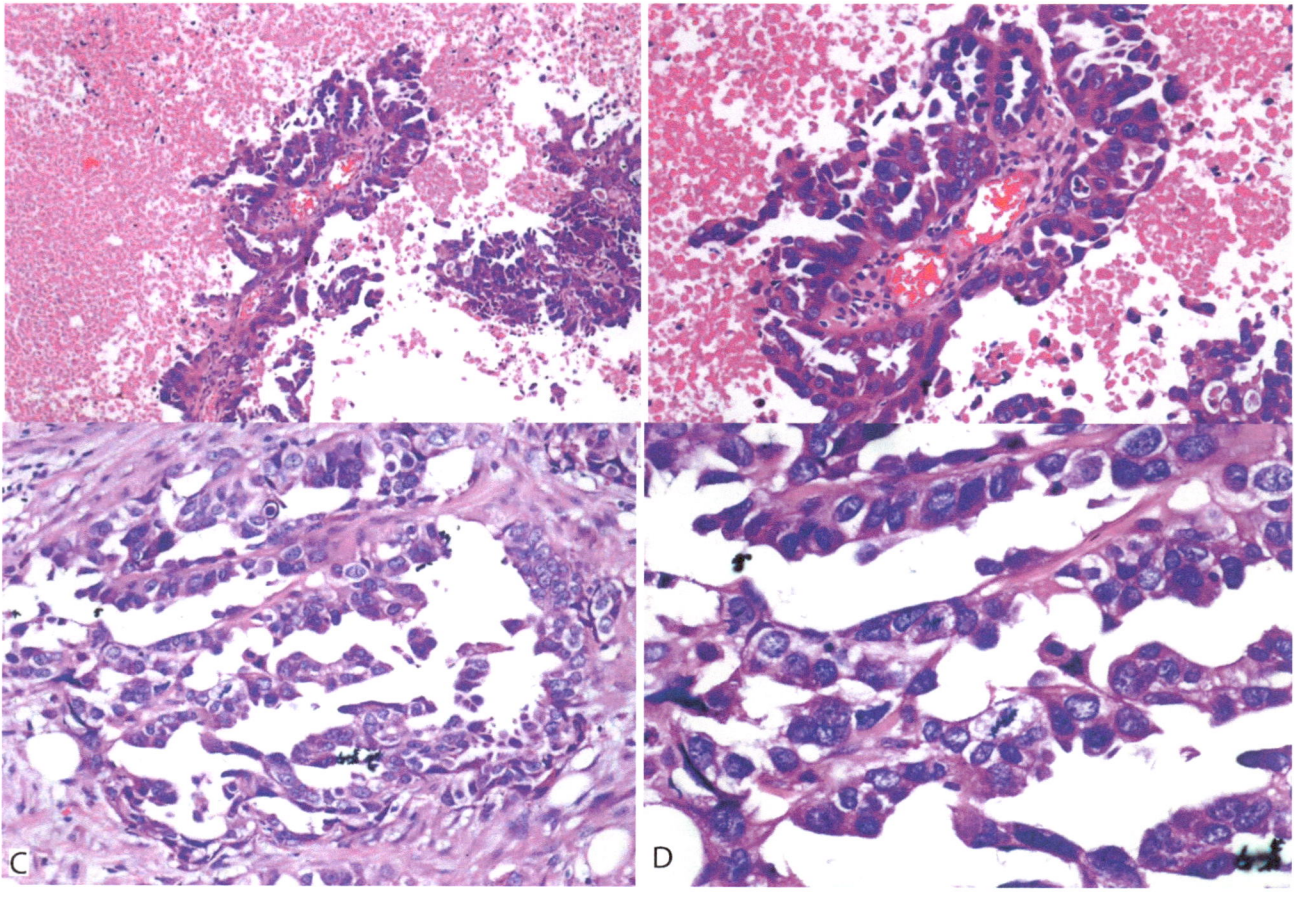

Figure 4 Serous papillary carcinoma of endometrium: (A,B) Scanner view; (C,D) Papillary pattern is evident

Serous Endometrial Cancers (SC) That Mimic Endometrioid Carcinomas (EC)

SC can exhibit cytologically high grade, architecturally well differentiated, tubulo-glandular morphology without an accompanying papillary growth pattern. Serous carcinomas can show glandular architecture in the form of gaping glands with ragged luminal contour and small papillary infoldings. It will be difficult to distinguish this form of SC from poorly differentiated endometrial adenocarcinoma.

In a recent study, a panel of immunostains has been employed to solve this problem 17. Approximately 75% to 90% of serous carcinoma (SC) cases express p53 in a strong and diffuse fashion (Figure 5 A-F). However, some cases of endometrioid carcinoma also express p53 but it is focal and weak staining. It may be noted, that immunohistochemistry shows lack of estrogen and progesterone receptors in SC as against positive ER PR receptors present in endometrioid adenocarcinoma.

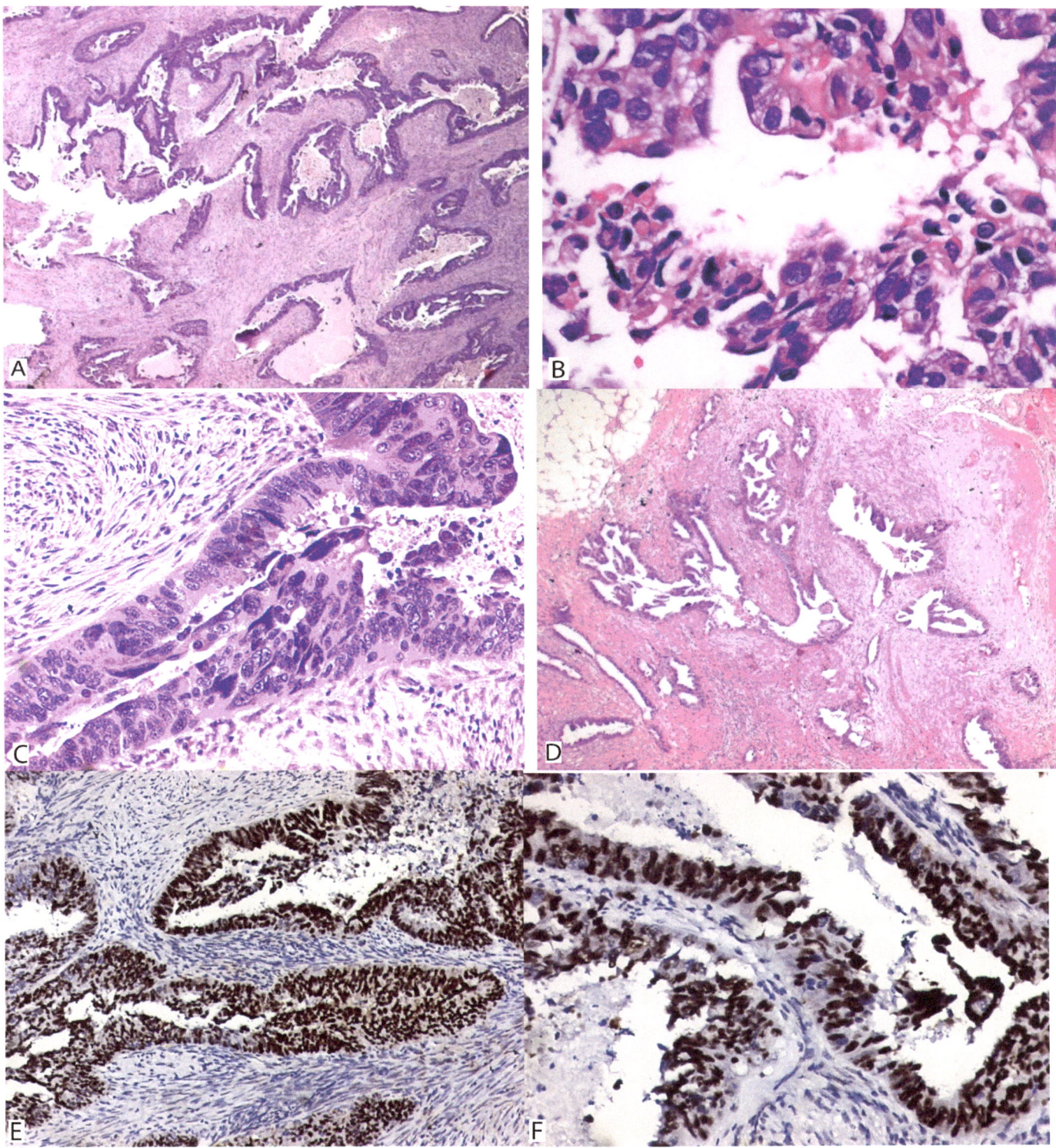

Figure 5 Endometrial adenocarcinoma arising in endometrial polyp (A) Serous papillary carcinoma of the endometrium; (B, C) papillary and glandular patterns with marked nuclear anaplasia in; (D) shows metastasis in omentum. (E, F) Strong and diffuse P53 nuclear positivity

Endometrial Intraepithelial Carcinoma (EIC)

EIC is a relatively recently described entity, defined as replacement of the uterine surface epithelium and/or underlying glands by high grade malignant epithelial cells and presents as the "in situ" phase of serous carcinoma (SC). Thus, it frequently coexists with uterine serous carcinoma (EC) and is hypothesized to be its precursor lesion. Wheelar et al 18 studied 8 cases of pure EIC and 13 cases of superficial serous carcinoma without myometrial or vascular invasion. The review demonstrated that the most important feature in assessing prognosis is the presence or absence of extra-uterine disease at presentation; 13 of 14 patients (93%) of EIC or SC confined to the uterus were disease free; whereas seven patients who presented with extra-uterine disease, even if only microscopic, were either dead or alive with disease. One report showed cases of EIC alone, who were found to have multiple, synchronous foci of extra-uterine serous carcinoma at presentation 19. Hysterectomy in all cases showed endometrial polyps with EIC but without invasive SC. P53 expression was observed in both EIC and peritoneal deposits of SC. Thus, finding of EIC in an endometrial curettage should prompt a thorough search of invasive carcinoma in uterus or extra uterine sites

Serous carcinoma arising in endometrial polyp

In a series of 97 cases of serous carcinoma of endometrium, 13 (13%) developed in an endometrial polyp 20. All primary tumors (except 1) were limited to the polyp but in 4 of 13 cases extra uterine disease was present. This indicates that if only a polypectomy or hysterectomy was performed, most cases of extra uterine disease would be missed. About 80 cases of SC with associated polyp have been published 20. Figure 5 (G, H, I) shows histological changes of polyp with hyperplastic and highly atypical endometrial glands. Figure 5 J reveals malignant glands exhibiting strong diffuse immunostaining with p53. The pathogenetic relationship of benign endometrial polyp and serous carcinoma (SC) has not been dealt with in the literature. It is not clear whether endometrial polyp has a precancerous role in the genesis of endometrial carcinoma.

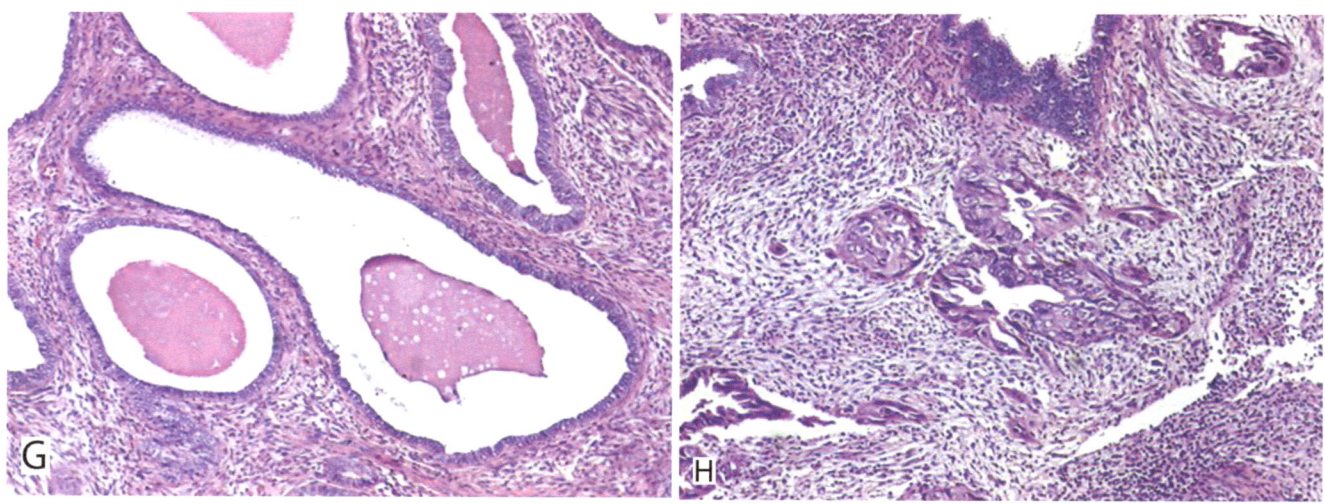

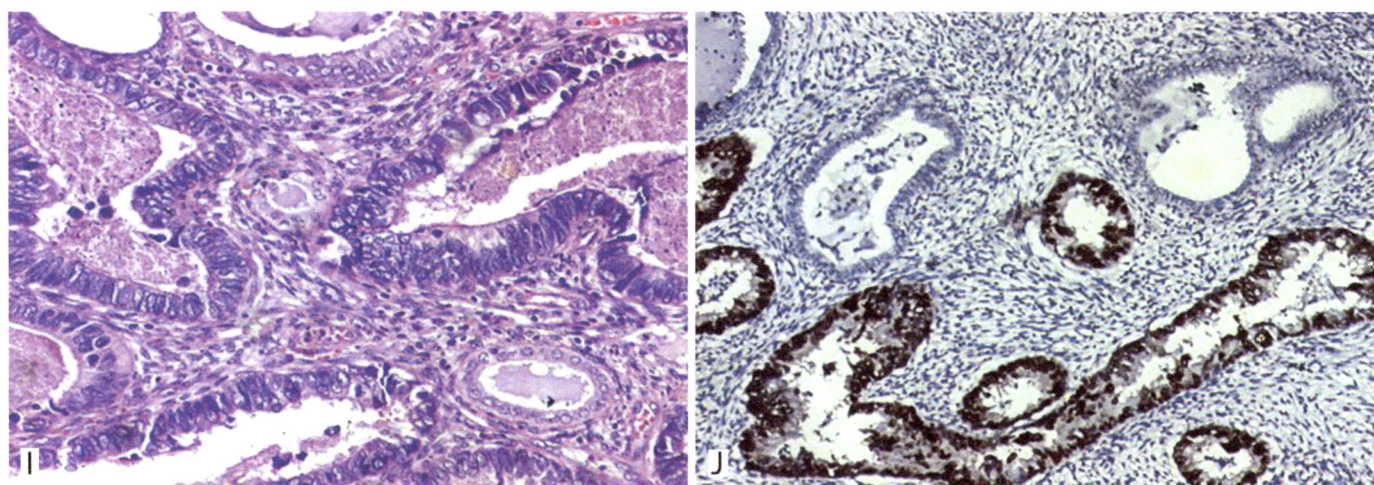

Figure 5 (G) Low power view of endometrial polyp; (H) a mixture of benign and atypical glands; (I) high power view of intraepithelial carcinoma (J) Strong and diffuse immunostaining for p53 in neoplastic glands, note negative immunostaining for benign glands for p53; the immunohistochemical findings above indicate that this is an intraepithelial serous carcinoma, arising in a polyp.

Prognosis

Serous carcinoma has a propensity of myometrial and lymphatic invasion. Hysterectomy specimen often discloses tumor in lymphatics in myometrium, cervix, broad ligament, fallopian tube and ovarian hilum. Serous carcinoma involves peritoneal surfaces of pelvis and abdomen quite early in the course of the disease and SC is understaged in about 40% of cases.

Data from Norway 21: The 5- and 10 year actuarial survival rates
For the entire group of 1977 endometrial adenocarcinomas: 73.1% and 61% respectively

Serous carcinoma (SC); 27% and 14% respectively
Intramucosal tumors: 89.6% and 82.5% respectively
Tumors infiltrating <half myometrium: 84% and 72.7% respectively
Tumors reaching serosa: 48.3% and 29.3% respectively
Tumors without vascular invasion: 83.5% and 61.1% respectively
Tumors with vascular invasion: 64.5% and 53.8% respectively

Clear Cell Carcinoma of Endometrium (CCC)

Definition

Clear cell carcinoma is an adenocarcinoma composed of glycogen filled clear or hobnail cells with high grade nuclear anaplasia and arrangement in solid, tubular or papillary patterns. It occurs usually in postmenopausal women and exhibits aggressive behavior. It was called mesonephric carcinoma in the past, because of its resemblance to renal cell carcinoma; and now its Mullerian origin is accepted 22. The histological features of endometrial CCC are similar to those seen in the ovarian, cervical and vaginal tumors that carry the same name.

Microscopic

CCC may exhibit solid, glandular, papillary or cystic patterns. The solid component is composed of contiguous sheets of clear cells with intermingled eosinophilic cells. The papillary glandular and cystic patterns are lined predominantly by hobnail-shaped cells with interspersed clear and eosinophilic cells. The tumor cells are usually large with clear or lightly eosinophilic cytoplasm and possess actively mitotic, pleomorphic and even bizarre nuclei. The presence of glycogen in tumor cells can be readily demonstrated with PAS stain and diastase digestion (Figure 6 A-D).

A putative precursor lesion for CCC has been described, being characterized by endometrial cells with clear and/or eosinophilic cytoplasm and varying degrees of nuclear anaplasia. These cells involve benign endometrial glands and surface epithelial cells adjacent to a clear cell carcinoma growth 23.

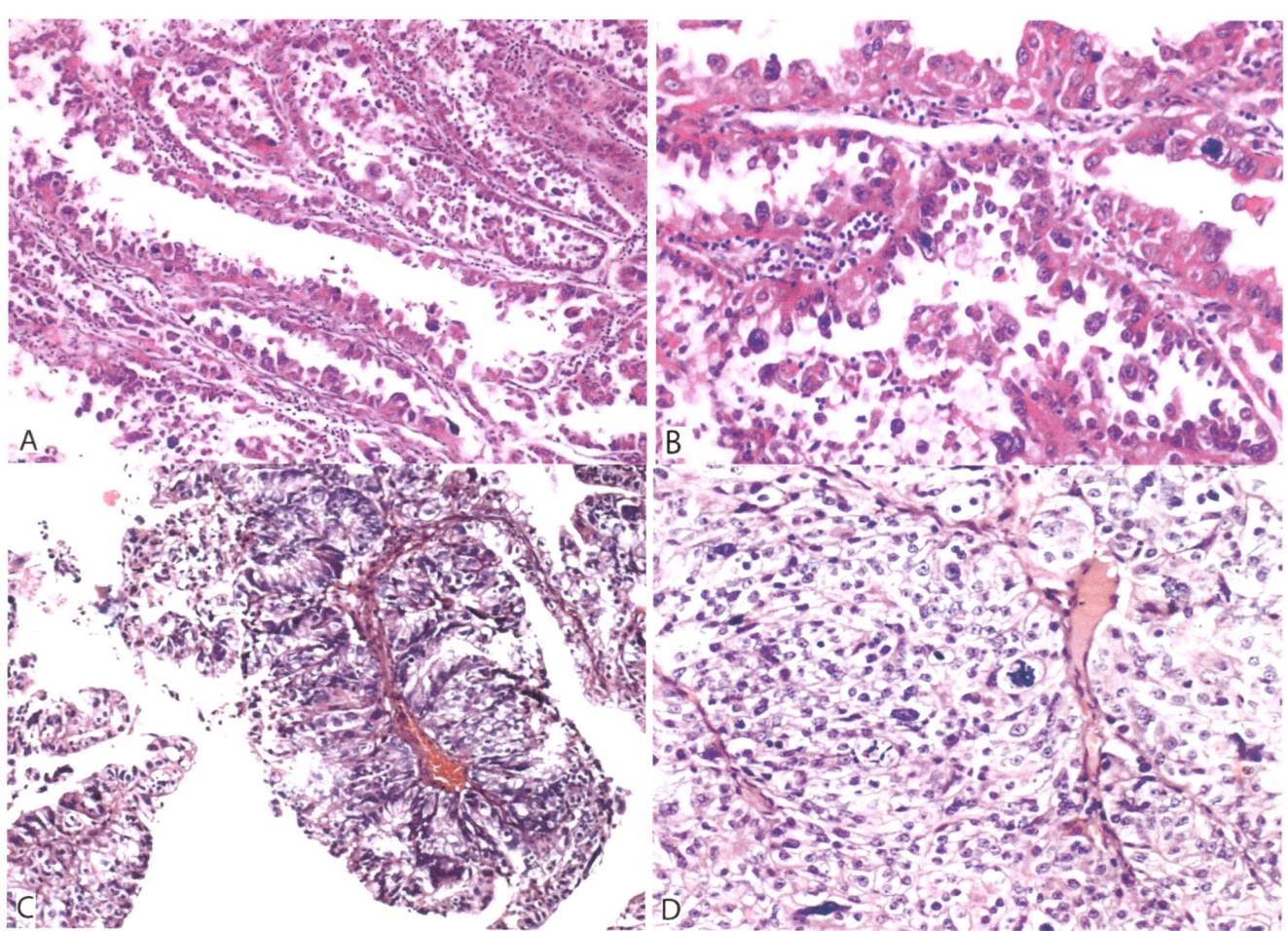

Figure 6 Clear cell carcinoma of the endometrium (A, B) showing tubular pattern and hobnailing; C-papillary pattern; D-high nuclear grade and clear cytoplasm

Differential Diagnosis

CCC should be differentiated from secretory carcinoma, serous carcinoma and yolk sac tumor. Distinction from serous carcinoma is based on architectural and cytoplasmic appearance rather than nuclear anaplasia because both tumors display high grade nuclear morphology. Differentiation from yolk sac tumor is not difficult because this tumor occurs in young patients, whereas CCC is a tumor of postmenopausal women. If there is histological overlap, presence of high serum AFP levels or its demonstration in the tumor tissue by immunohistochemistry will be diagnostic of yolk sac tumor.

Prognosis

An assessment of the clinical stage and depth of myometrial invasion are very useful in predicting the prognosis. In a series of 181 cases treated for CCC the 5-and 10 year actuarial survival rates for all stages were 43% and 39%, respectively, in a study from Norway 24. These survival rates appear rather low but attest to the aggressive nature of the tumor. In one recent study of 50 cases of CCC, however, 5-year progression free survival for the entire cohort was 61% 25.

Endometrial Adenocarcinoma in Women under 40 years of Age

Endometrial carcinoma is predominantly a disease of postmenopausal women. It is relatively rare in women younger than 40 years of age, accounting for only 2.1% to 14.4% of cases, most of whom wish to preserve their fertility 26. The common reported risk factors of endometrial cancer are anovulatory cycles associated with polycystic ovary syndrome, hypertension, diabetes, and obesity 27. It has been observed that the majority of cases of endometrial adenocarcinoma in younger women are of endometrioid type, well differentiated (Figure 7)) and occurring at an early stage with a superficial invasion (Stage I). These carcinomas have good prognosis with survival rate of >93% at five-years 28.

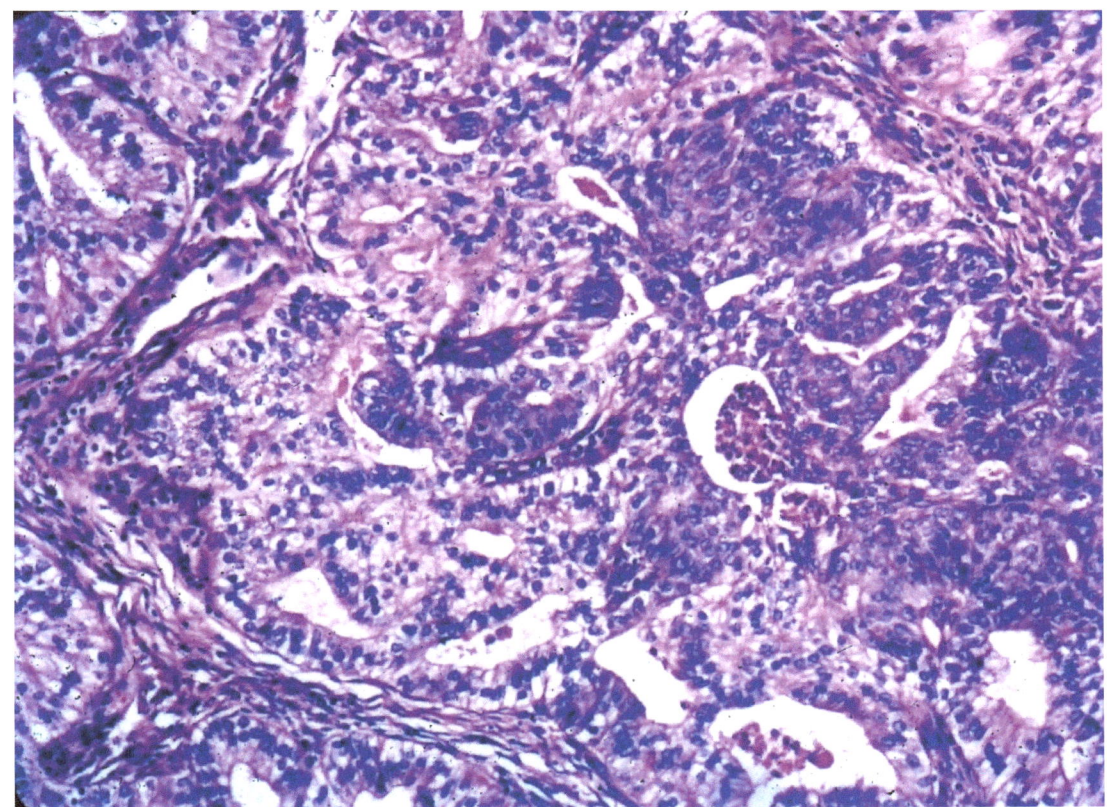

Figure 7 Endometrioid adenocarcinoma in an infertile woman, who had diagnostic endometrial curettage

The case illustrated in Figure 7 was treated with high dose progesterone, which produced partial regression with secretory changes. After some attempts at inducing ovulation the patient did not conceive and finally hysterectomy with bilateral salpingo-oophorectomy was carried out.

The standard treatment for endometrial carcinoma is total abdominal hysterectomy and bilateral salpingo-oophorectomy. However, there is a therapeutic alternative for young women wishing to become pregnant in future. There are reports of women 40 years or younger (<40), who had low grade and low stage endometrial carcinoma and who responded to hormonal manipulations followed by regression of carcinoma and occurrence of successful pregnancy in some. In a literature survey of 21 reports with endometrial carcinoma under 40 years of age, there were
58 child births among 130 treated patients 26 27, 28, 29. The most important factor for conservative treatment is selecting the "ideal patient", who should have following characteristics 30:

Well differentiated adenocarcinoma in stage 1
There should be no myometrial invasion as seen on MRI
3) Absence of suspicious pelvic nodes
4) Absence of synchronous ovarian tumors
5) The patient understands and accepts that this is not a standard treatment,
6) She should be willing to complete the follow-up protocol

It has been suggested that a large multicenter trial of fertility-preserving treatment is warranted for nulliparous young patients with well selected Stage I, Grade 1, endometrial adenocarcinoma31 Figure 7shows an endometrioid adenocarcinoma in an infertile woman, who had diagnostic endometrial curettage

Malignant Mixed Mullerian Tumors (MMMT)

The name malignant mixed Mullerian tumor is derived from observations of the embryonic female genitalia during the 6th week of embryogenesis. Epithelial and mesenchymal structures arise or are induced from the development of Mullerian ducts. In males, anti-Mullerian hormone secreted by the Sertoli cells of the testis causes rapid regression of the ducts. However, in females these ducts give rise to fallopian tube, uterus, cervix and proximal vagina 32.

Definition

Uterine MMMT is rare, highly aggressive, rapidly progressing, histologically biphasic neoplasm associated with a poor prognosis that has not significantly improved in the past 30 years despite advances in imaging and adjuvant therapy. It is composed of epithelial and mesenchymal elements and believed to arise from a monoclonal origin 32.

Synonyms

Malignant mixed mesodermal tumor, metaplastic carcinoma and carcinosarcoma are the terms reported in the literature and currently carcinosarcoma is the preferred designation 33.

Clinical Findings

The tumor occurs predominantly in postmenopausal women of low parity and the presenting features include abdominal pain, bowel symptoms and weight loss. The tumors are detected in decreasing frequency in the uterine corpus, cervix, vagina, ovaries and fallopian tubes 34. At the time of diagnosis, majority (70%) of these patients have tumor spread beyond the genital organs. The pattern of spread is primarily to the peritoneum, omentum and regional lymph nodes. Apart from fallopian tube and ovary, the tumor has been reported from many extra genital sites in the abdomen.

Gross

The tumors present as a large (average 15 cm), soft, and polypoid mass involving the endometrium and myometrium, sometimes protruding through the external cervical os. Sectioned surface shows foci of necrosis and prominent hemorrhages and necrosis (Figure 8 A-D).

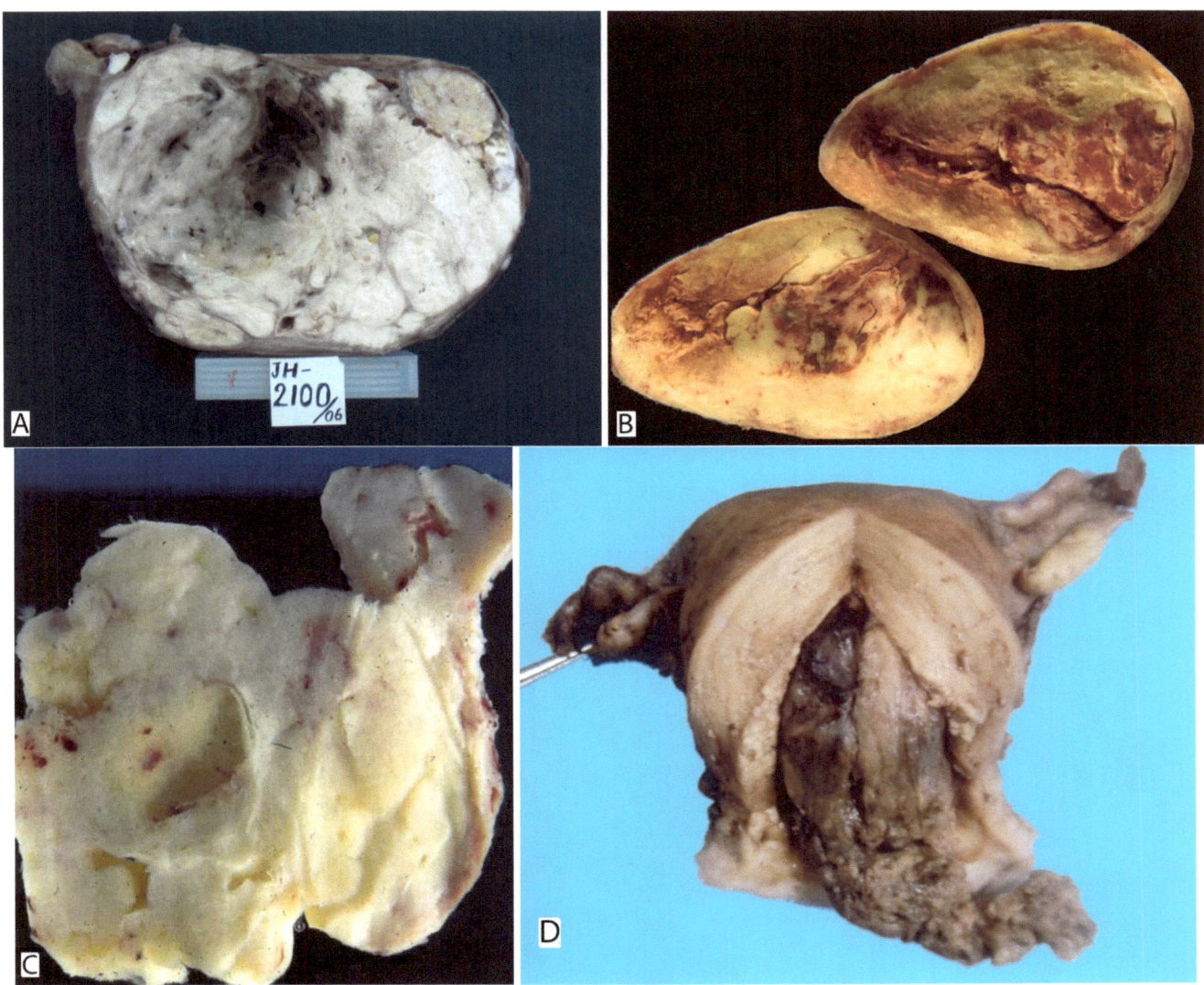

Figure 8 Gross: Different faces of MMMT (A) large whitish circumscribed tumor occupying uterine corpus completely, note focal necrosis and hemorrhages; (B) well circumscribed fundal mass with extensive hemorrhages and necrosis; (C) rather soft fleshy whitish tumor with punctuate hemorrhages and focal yellowish mottling; (D) Large polypoid necrotic and hemorrhagic tumor protruding through the external os of the cervix.

Microscopic

MMMTs are characterized by unique biphasic morphology, a tumor composed of both epithelial and mesenchymal elements. The epithelial component is often a high grade carcinoma such as papillary, serous or endometrioid (Figure 9 A, B). It may be composed of squamous cell carcinoma, basaloid squamous carcinoma, adenocarcinoma, adenosquamous carcinoma or undifferentiated carcinoma. The mesenchymal elements may be homologous undifferentiated sarcoma (Figure 9 C) or heterologous including chondrosarcoma, rhabdomyosarcoma (Figure 10 A-C), osteosarcoma or liposarcoma.

Some cases of MMMT show marked anaplasia in both carcinomatous and sarcomatous components (Figure 11 A-F). About 17 % of reported MMMTs reveal neuroendocrine differentiation and these cases exhibit more aggressive behavior 35. Other unusual histological features include melanocytic, yolk sac tumor or mesonephric pattern 36, 37. In large majority of cases histological diagnosis of MMMT can be readily made and immunohistochemistry is not necessary. However, in difficult cases with a differential diagnosis, positive CK 7 with negative CK 20 and presence of CD10 in the stromal cells provide immunohistochemical evidence of a Mullerian origin.

It has been reported that the epithelial component of MMMTS invades lymphatic/vascular spaces and metastasize, whereas the spindle cell component has limited metastatic potential, if any. Since the behavior is dictated by the epithelial element, it is suggested that malignant mixed Mullerian tumors of uterus should be classified as carcinomas rather than sarcomas. This has great therapeutic implications since chemotherapy protocols are different for carcinomas and sarcomas 38.

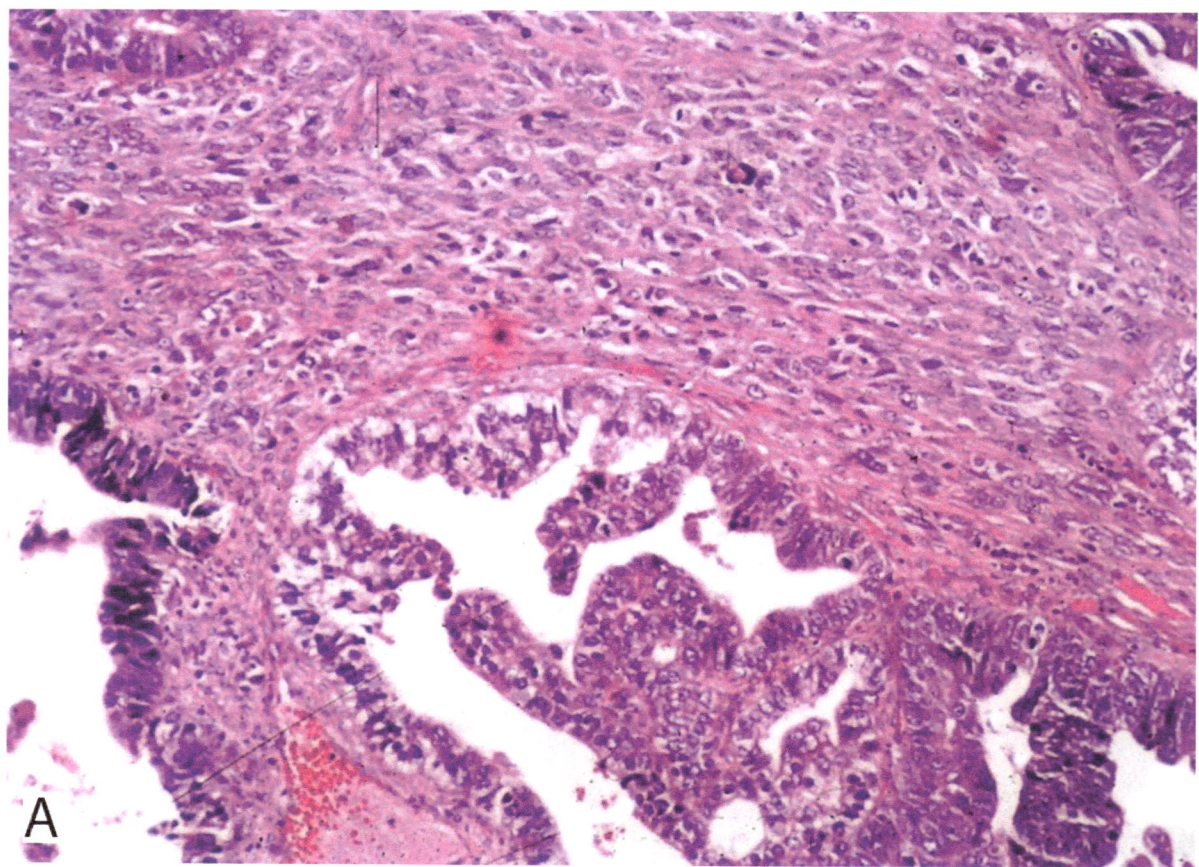

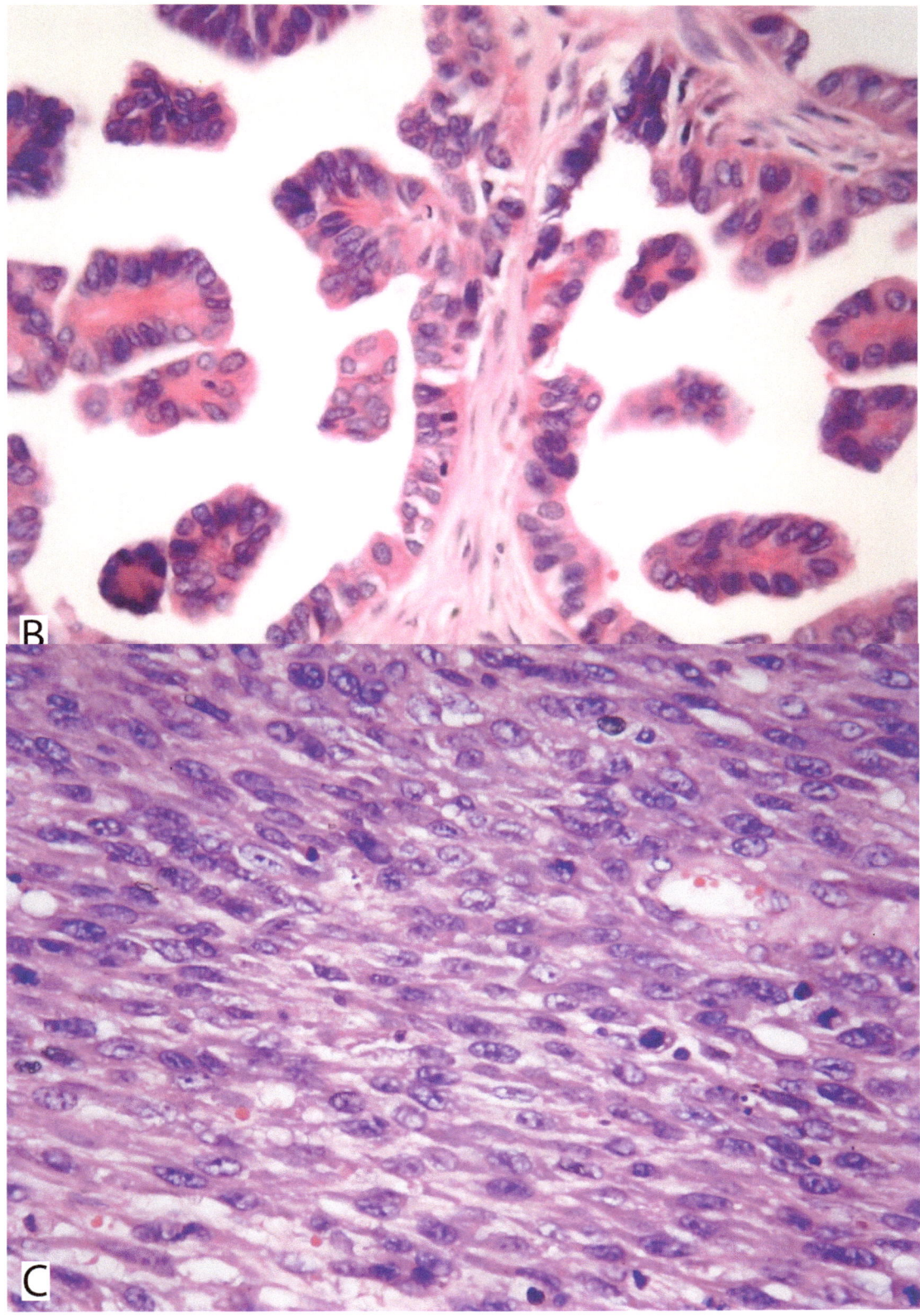

Fig 9 MMMT: (A, B) predominant glandular component; (C) monomorphic homologous high grade sarcomatous component

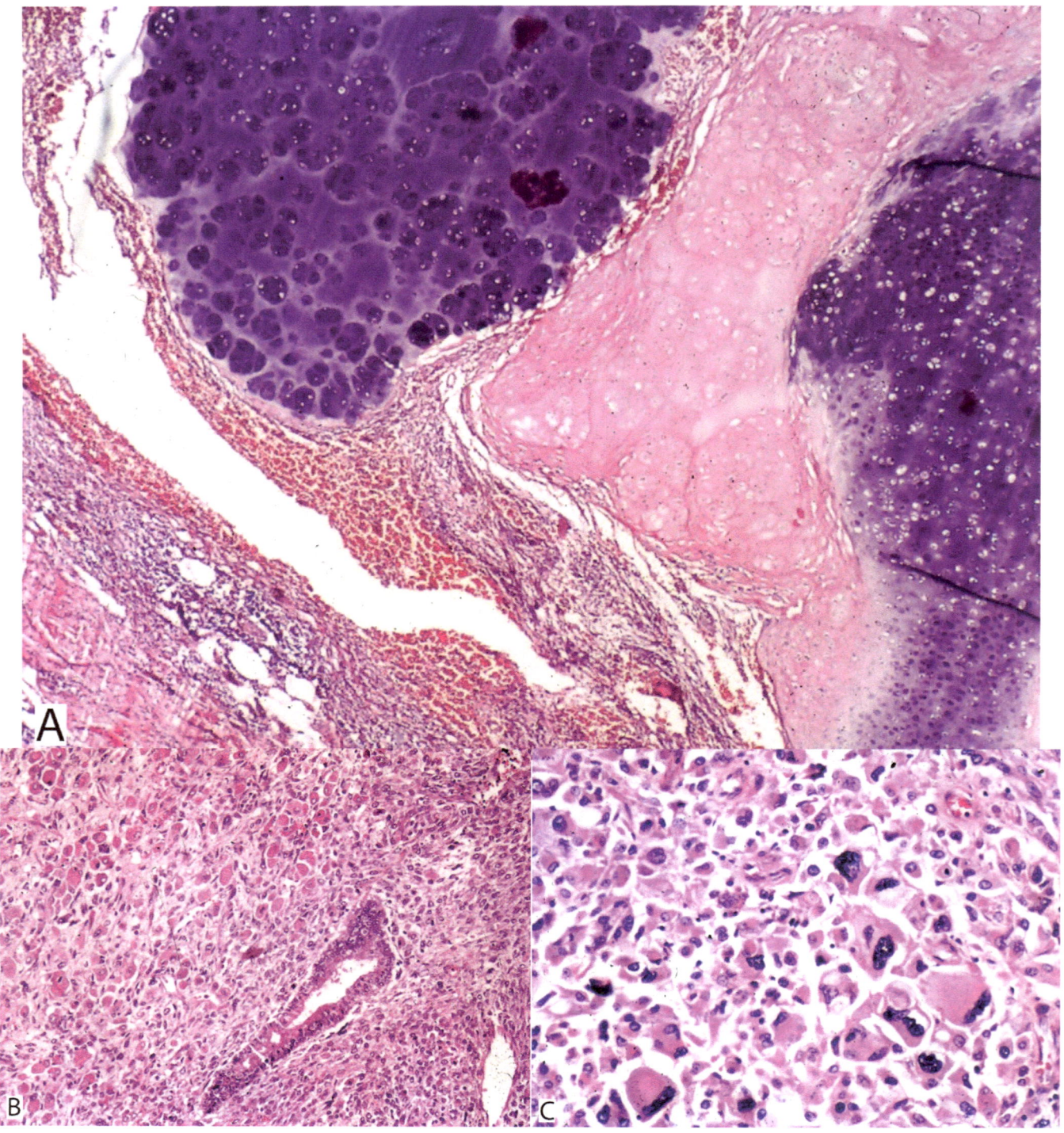

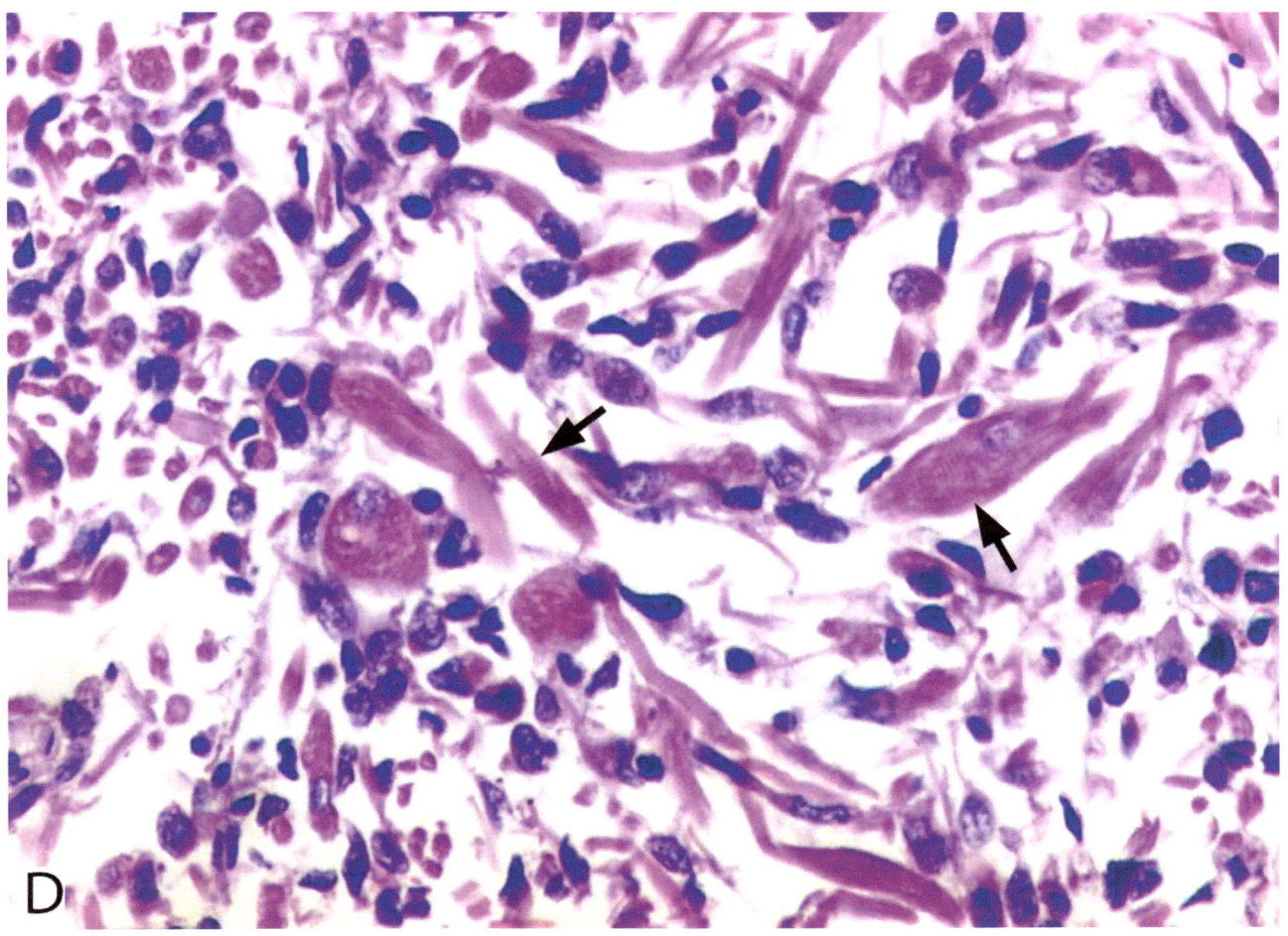

Figure 10 MMMT heterologous elements: (A) chondroid islands; (B, C) rhabdomyoblastic differentiation (D)a more vivid rhabdomyoblastic feature from another case, note cross striations (arrows)

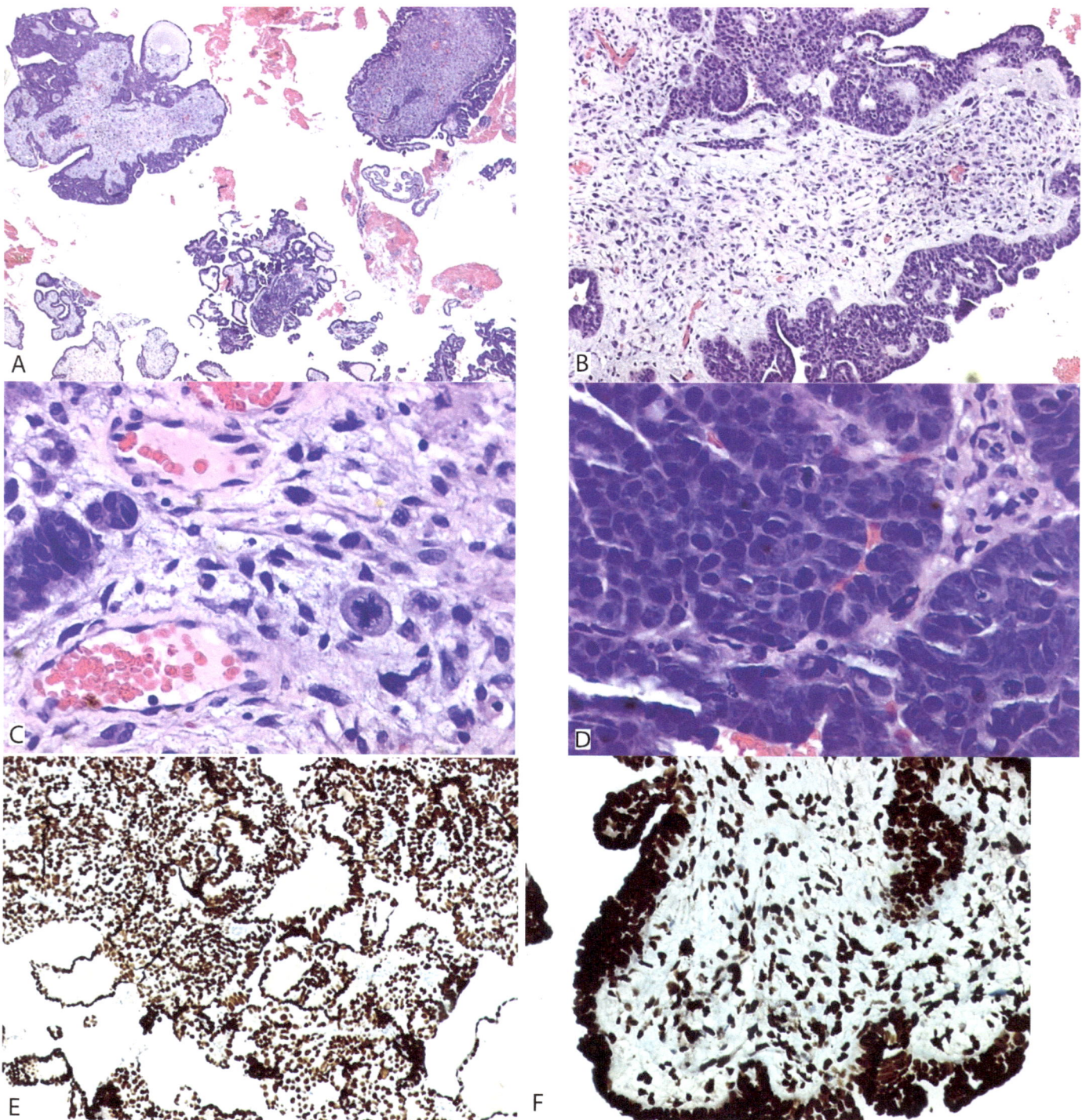

Figure 11 MMMT: (A-D) Carcinosarcoma: both components are anaplastic; (E, F) P53 shows strong nuclear positivity

Prognosis

Over the past 30 years despite evolving and advancing therapeutic regimens, prognosis remains poor, with no significant improvements in survival or recurrence rate. Assessment of prognosis is difficult because a large number of publications are case reports and only a handful of articles are reported as series. Some of these reports often lack in information on stage stratification.

MMMTs are often diagnosed at an advanced stage which contributes to the poor 5 year overall survival rate of 35%. The disease free survival rate of patients with stage I MMMTs were worse compared with stage I high grade endometrial carcinoma The 3-yrs overall survival rates are 45% versus 93% in patients with heterologous compared with homologous stage I MMMT.39

Five year survival rates in early uterine carcinosarcoma (FIGO Stages I & II) are between 30%-46%, and 0% to 10% in advanced cancers (Stage III & IV) 32

Mullerian Adenosarcoma (MA)

Definition

The term Mullerian adenosarcoma (MA) was introduced by Clement and Scully in 1974 to designate an uncommon variant of Mullerian mixed tumor of the uterus, characterized by a benign but occasionally atypical glandular component and a sarcomatous stromal component, which is usually low grade 40.

In the last 30 years since the first description of this tumor, approximately 300 cases have been reported in the world literature.

Clinical findings

The patients present with abnormal vaginal bleeding, enlarged uterus and polypoid mass protruding through the external os. Usually, preoperative diagnosis of adenosarcoma cannot be arrived at. It is a rare neoplasm typically arising in the endometrium, but has also been reported in the ovary, cervix and extra pelvic sites 41.

Gross

The tumor typically grows as a polypoid mass arising from the endometrial mucosa and filling the uterine cavity It very rarely involves the myometrium. The sectioned surface of the mass reveals tan brown soft to firm focally hemorrhagic tissue.

Microscopic

The distinguishing feature is the fact that epithelial (glandular) component is benign and cellular stromal component is akin to endometrial stroma. The stroma is abundant, cellular and exhibits hyperchromatic nuclei (Figure 12 A). At low power (scanner) the tumor has a leafy appearance (Figure 12 B) indistinguishable from that of phylloides tumor of breast.

Isolated glands, dilated or compressed into thin slits, are dispersed through the mesenchymal component. The presence of stromal condensation surrounding glands or clefts is a typical finding of this tumor. The mesenchymal element is a low grade homologous stromal sarcoma containing varying amount of fibrous tissue and muscle. It has been estimated that about two mitosis per 10 HPF occurs, usually located in the hypercellularity stromal cuffs around the glands. Heterologous components like skeletal muscle, cartilage, adipocytes etc. are encountered in approximately 10% to 15% of cases. Vaginal or pelvic recurrence in approximately 25% to30% of cases occurs at 5 years and is associated almost exclusively with myometrial invasion and sarcomatous overgrowth 41, 42, 43

Immunohistochemical studies show variable expression of ER, PR, CD10, SMA and desmin in the typical Mullerian adenosarcoma 44. This immunophenotype resembles that of endometrial stromal tumors. Clement and Scully described in 1989, 10 cases of MA of the uterus with sarcomatous overgrowth, all having an identifiable component of classical MA but overgrown by homologous or heterologous high grade sarcoma. These tumors did not express ER, PR and CD10 unlike MA, reflecting the "dedifferentiation" of the stromal component in MA with sarcomatous overgrowth. An immunohistochemical study revealed that CD 10 expression is not restricted to ESS but can be positive in MMMT and MA as well as in a variety of uterine tumors including high-grade leiomyosarcoma and rhabdomyosarcoma. CD 10 might be one of the characteristics of Mullerian system-derived neoplastic mesenchymal cells 45.

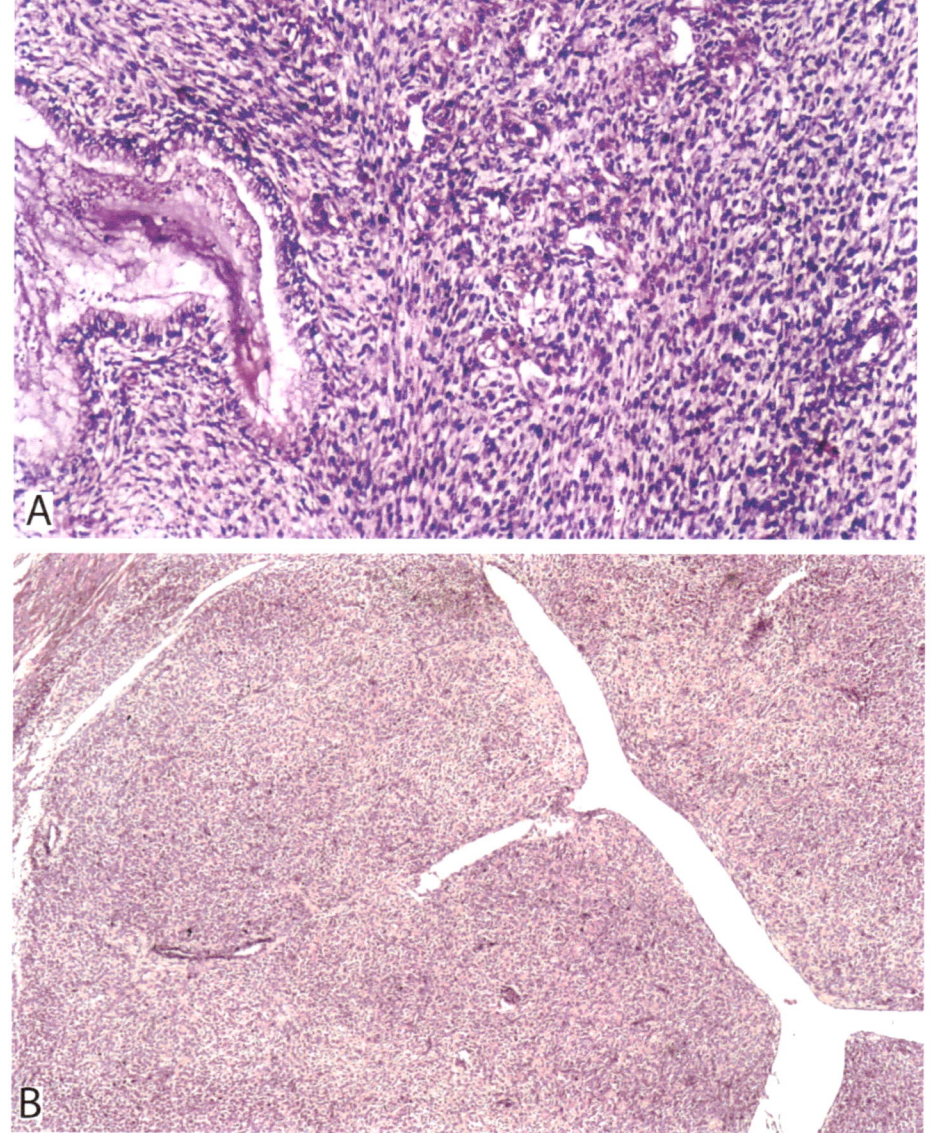

Fig 12 Adenosarcoma (A) A benign glands surrounded by copious sarcomatous stroma with excess cellularity and hyperchromatic nuclei; (B) Low power view showing abundant low grade sarcomatous stroma and compressed distorted benign glands, note resemblance to histology of benign phyllodes tumor

Prognosis

Unlike MMMTs, most adenosarcomas are tumors of low malignant potential. Adenosarcoma has always been regarded as a low grade neoplasm and yet it recurs in 25% to 40% of cases. Recurrent tumor is usually seen in vagina or pelvis, often a number of years postoperatively. Death from tumor occurs in about 10% of patients. The presence of myometrial invasion and sarcomatous overgrowth has been shown to be consistently associated with poor prognosis 42.

Endometrial Stromal Tumor (EST)

Definition

Endometrial stromal sarcomas are tumors composed of cells resembling those of proliferative phase endometrial stroma. The tumors are rare and show great morphological variation, indolent growth and variable biological behavior.

The traditional classification of ESS into low-grade and high-grade categories has fallen out of favor and high-grade tumors without recognizable evidence of a definite endometrial stromal phenotype are now termed undifferentiated endometrial stromal sarcomas instead of high-grade ESS. Undifferentiated endometrial stromal sarcoma (UES) represents a high grade sarcoma that lacks specific differentiation and bears no histological resemblance to endometrial stroma, and therefore the term ESS is now best considered restricted to neoplasms that were formerly referred to as low grade ESS 46, 47.

Current Classification of ESS

1) Endometrial Stromal Nodule
2) Low-grade Endometrial Stromal Sarcoma
3) Undifferentiated Endometrial Stromal Sarcoma (a high grade sarcoma with no resemblance to endometrial stroma]

Low Grade Endometrial Stroma Sarcoma

Clinical Features

A proper clinical diagnosis is difficult and in most cases the diagnosis is confirmed after a hysterectomy for presumed benign diagnosis. The most common clinical manifestations are uterine enlargement, abnormal vaginal bleeding and at times pelvic pain.

Gross

It presents as a multi nodular growth or a solitary well defined and predominantly intramural mass (Figure 13 A, B) and histologically extensive permeation of the myometrium is always present (Figure 13 C); extension to serosa is seen in about 50% of cases. Endometrium may be involved and the presence of ESS in the curetted material may be missed. Sectioned surface of the tumor appears yellow or tan and has a softer consistency than the usual leiomyoma.

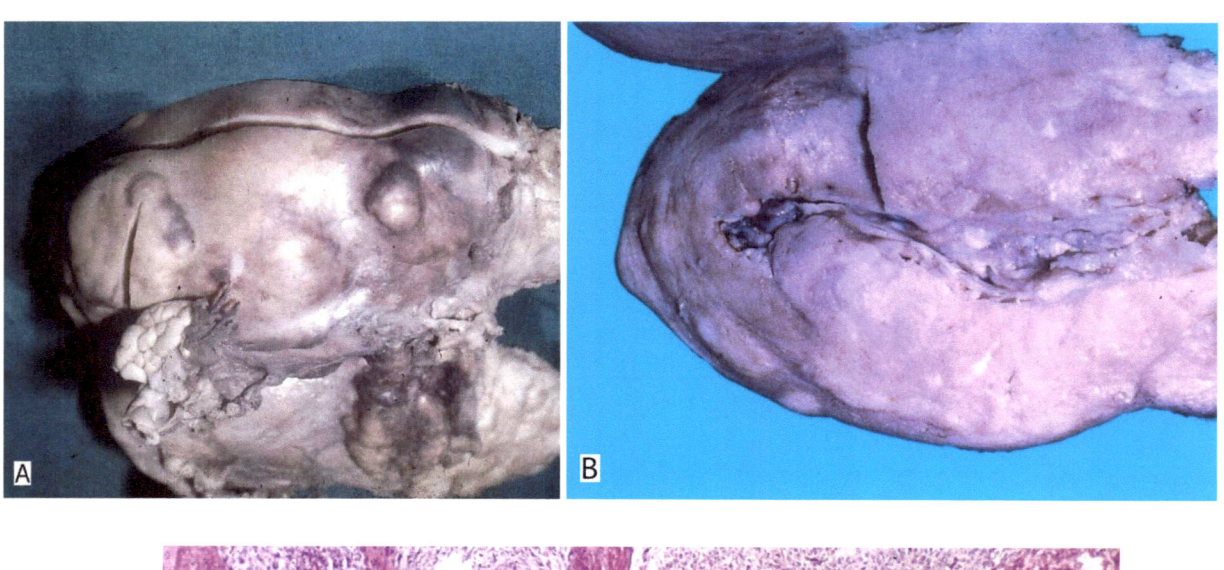
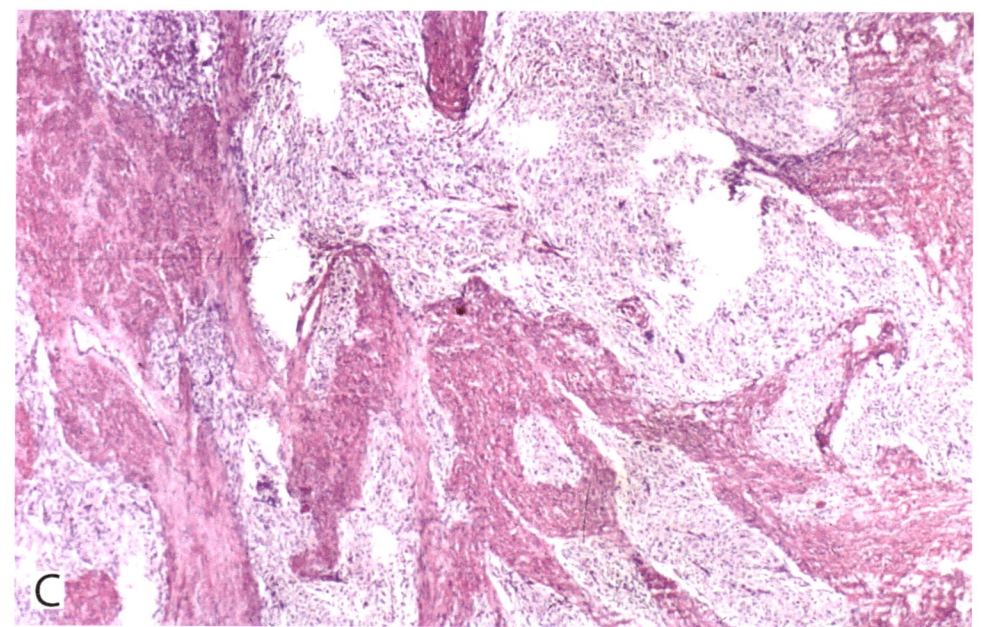

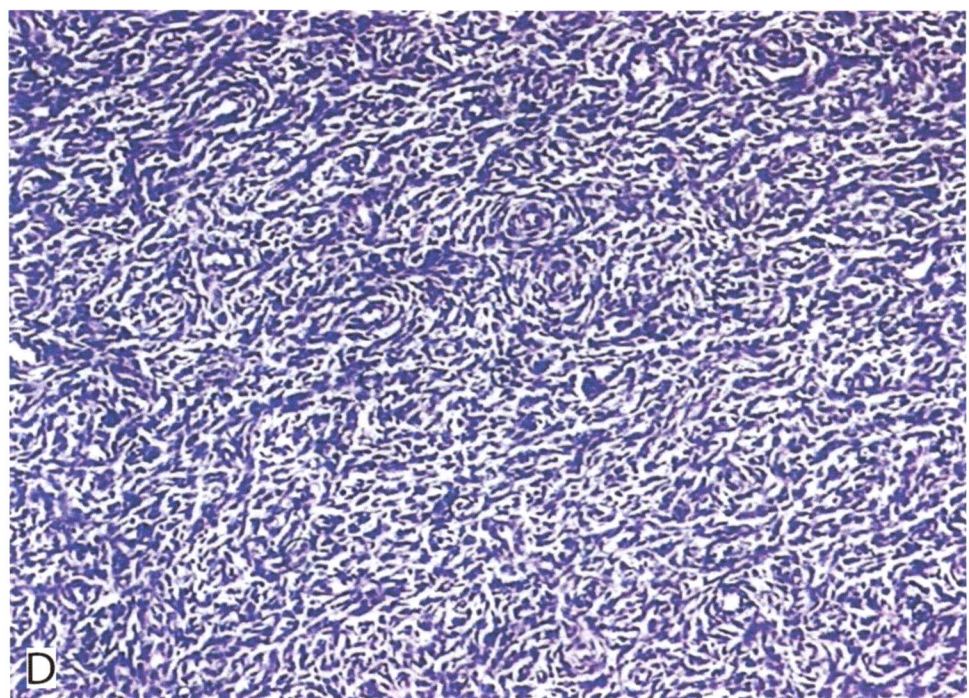

Figure 13 Endometrial Stroma Sarcoma (A) multicentric uterine nodules are seen indistinguishable from fibroids; (B) hypertrophic myometrium containing small widely scattered whitish nodules; (C) broad bands of ESS cells randomly infiltrating and dissecting the myometrium; (D) close up of ESS (from another case)showing small oval to short spindly cells in cellular sheets interrupted by small thin walled vessels. Thanks are due to Dr Santosh Menon Associate Professor and Pathologist, Tata Memorial Hospital, Mumbai for contributing Figure 13 (D)

Microscopic

The tumor is densely cellular and consists of closely packed oval to round cells, supported by a rich network of small thin walled vessels (Figure 13 D). In many cases, cellular plugs of the tumor tissue are seen in the myometrial lymphatics, which led to the now abandoned term "endolymphatic stromal myosis" (Figure 14 A, B). The cells have scanty cytoplasm, round nuclei and inconspicuous nucleoli. No significant atypia or pleomorphism is present. Mitotic activity may not be discernible or may be found in about <5 per 10 HPF. Higher mitotic activity is encountered in some cases but this does not influence the biological behavior. In the low-grade ESS, extra uterine involvement occurs in about a third of cases. The extension appears as worm like plugs within lymphatics and blood vessels of the ovary (Figure 14 C), tube and broad ligament. In another case of endometrial sarcoma, the tumor is quite cellular and shows mitotic activity (Figure 14 D). CD 10 immunohistochemical staining shows sharply defined stromal sarcoma with adjacent unstained myometrium (Figure 14 E, F).

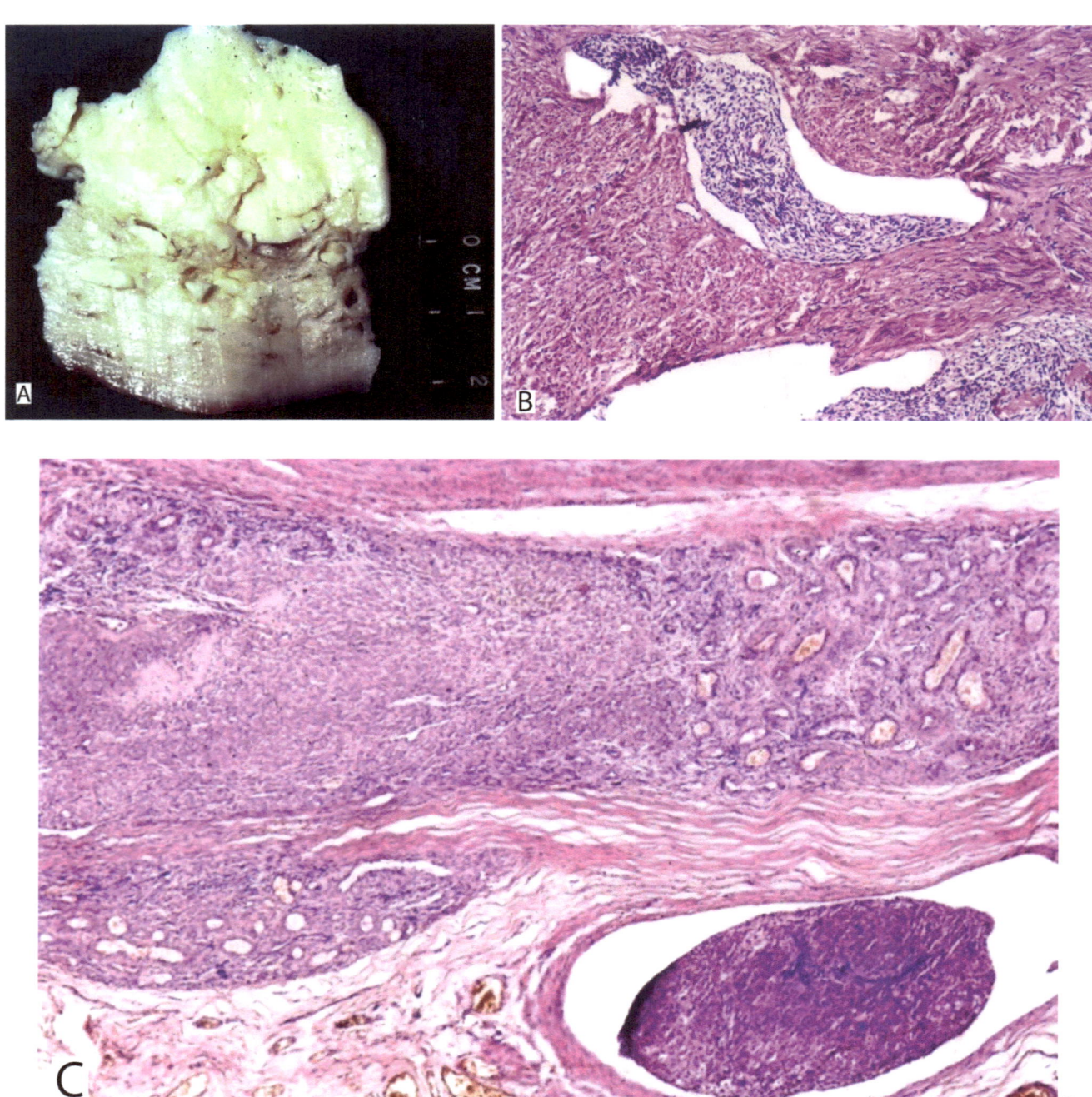

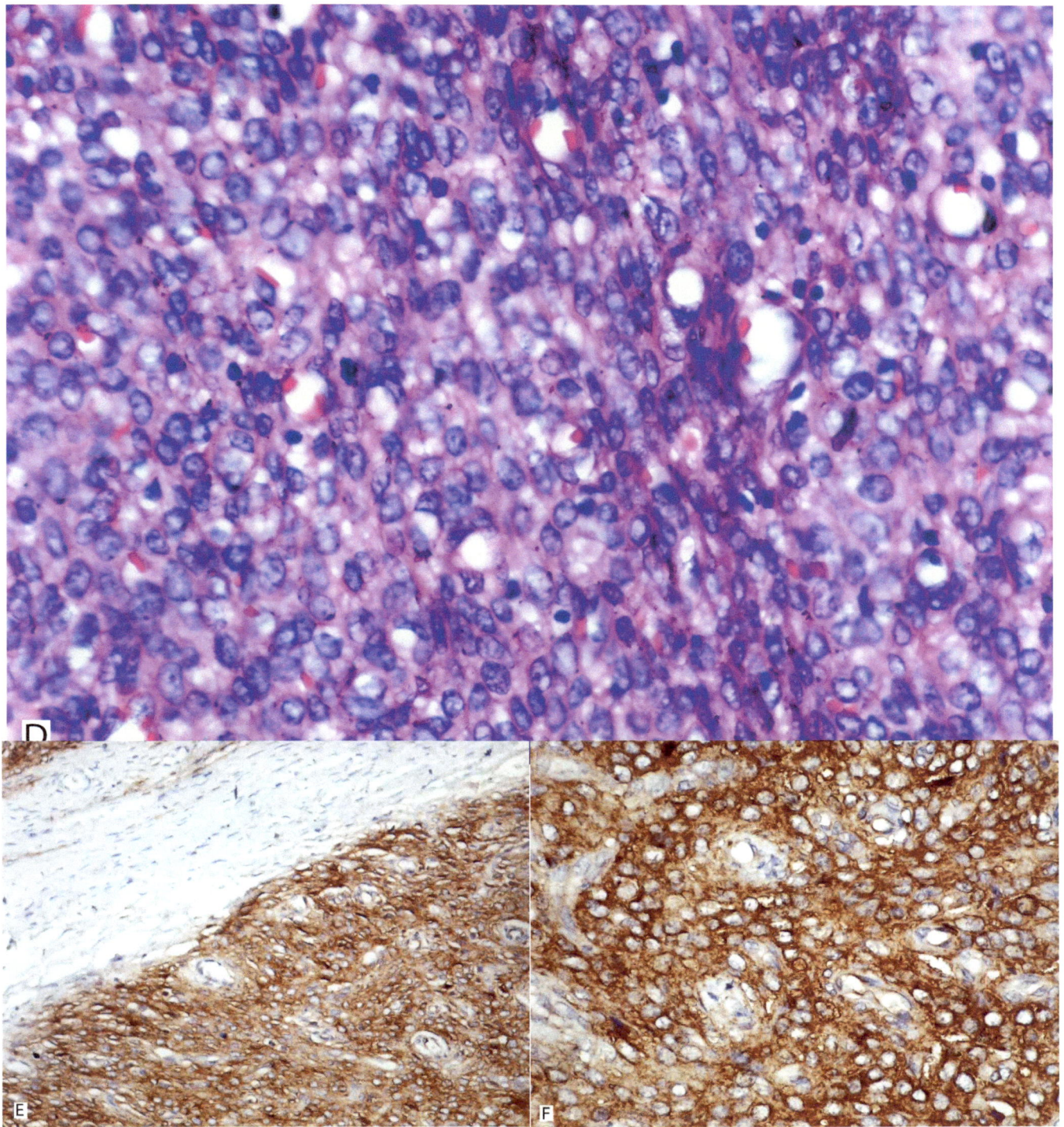

Figure 14 (A) solid growth in the endometrium and multiple small whitish nodules in the spaces in the myometrium; (B) dilated sinuous lymphatic spaces containing elongated strips of neoplastic endometrial stromal cells; (C) a large vessel plugged with ESS tumor nodule; near the ovarian hilum; (D) ESS, H&E; (E) CD 10 immunostained stromal sarcoma and surrounding unstained myometrium; (F) closeup of stromal tumor cells stained with CD 10

Immunohistochemistry

The most common lesion to be differentiated from ESS is benign or malignant smooth muscle tumor. The smooth muscle tumors express h Caldesmon, desmin and oxytocin receptors while CD10 and inhibin expression is a feature of ESS, which is almost always positive for both estrogen and progesterone receptors 46.

Prognosis

Low-grade ESS has a favorable prognosis with 5- and 10- year survival rates of up to 100%. However, recurrence is not uncommon and tends to be limited to the pelvis. Some patients may develop metastases after long tumor-free intervals. The most commonly affected site is the lung with reported incidence ranging from 7% to 28% 48.

The metastasis of endometrial sarcoma can occur 10 to 15 years after successful surgical therapy and then it is very difficult to make an accurate histological diagnosis of metastatic pulmonary lesion. The differential diagnoses for metastasis include sclerosing hemangioma, carcinoid tumor, lymphangioleiomyomatosis, hemangiopericytoma, synovial sarcoma, solitary fibrous tumor etc. Pulmonary metastases of ESS are associated with an excellent prognosis. Previous series of low-grade ESS reported an overall survival of 100% at 5 and 10 years, indicating that development of pulmonary metastases have little effect on survival.

In cases of metastasis to liver (an exceptional occurrence), resection of the disease has been documented. This is not unlike hepatic resection in neuroendocrine tumors of GI tract and pancreas. The experts have recommended resection of liver metastasis even if there are more sites of extra uterine disease, which are resectable 49. ESS is indeed an indolent low grade tumor but can disseminate well beyond the pelvis; an anecdotal case of vascular permeation with intracardiac metastasis has been reported recently 50.

Endometrial Stromal Nodule

It is characterized by a well delineated expansive margin and the cellular component is histologically identical to that of low-grade ESS. The tumor mass may fill the endometrial cavity and shows tan-yellow to brown sectioned surface. A fair number of these lesions occur exclusively in the myometrium with no connection to the endometrium. The interface of the solitary nodule and adjoining myometrium is always well defined (Figure 15 A-D)

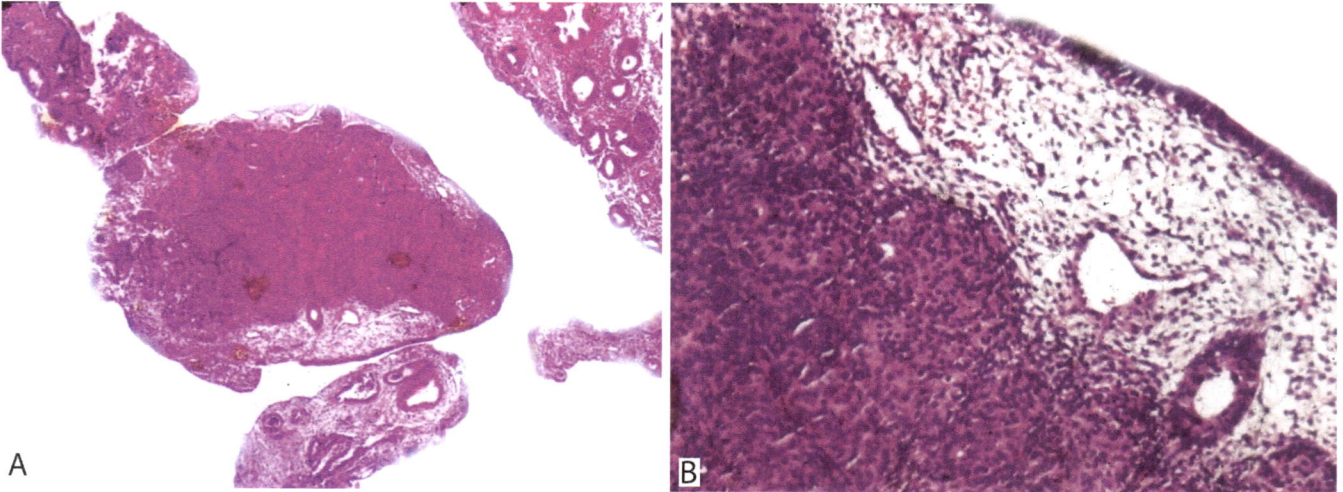

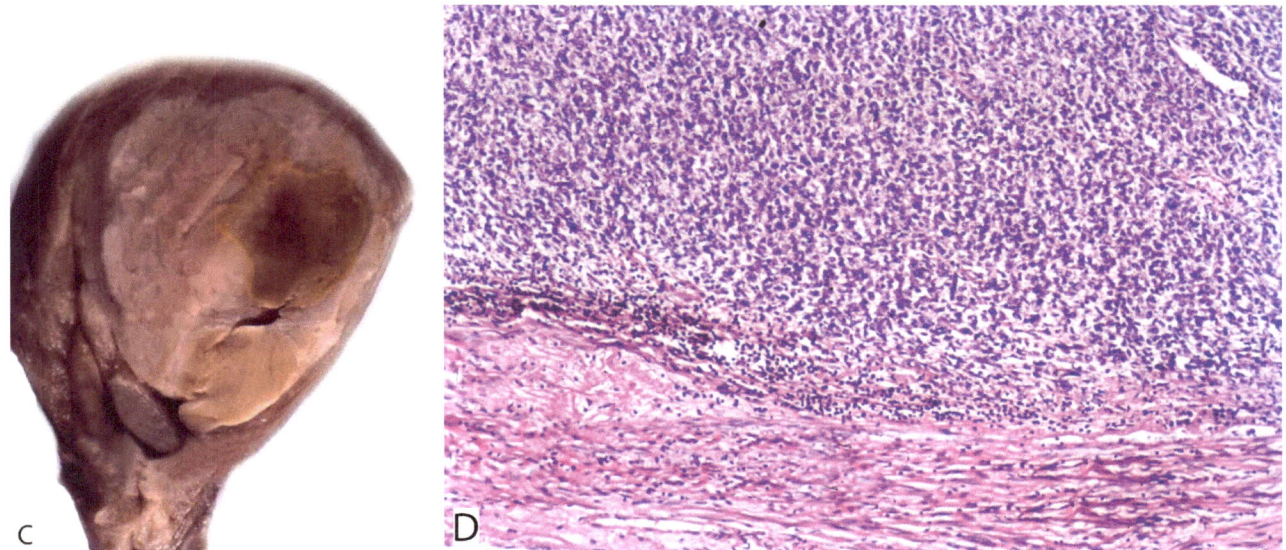

Figure 15 (A&B) Part of an endometrial stromal nodule seen in the curetted endometrial tissue; C- Endometrial cavity is dilated and filled with a sharply demarcated grey yellowish brown tumor (D) The interface of tumor nodule and myometrium is well defined.

In large series of 117 endometrial stromal neoplasms, there were 109 cases of ESS and 8 cases of stromal nodules for which, the differential diagnosis includes low grade ESS and cellular leiomyoma. The latter shows interdigitating smooth muscle bundles, large thick walled vessels and expression of immunoreactivity with desmin and h Caldesmon, which are diagnostic of smooth muscle lineage. Absence of CD 10 reactivity in leiomyoma will readily distinguish it from ESS 51. The cellular composition of endometrial stromal nodule is similar to that of low grade ESS. But stromal nodule is always sharply defined and ESS always infiltrates the myometrium or even beyond the confines of uterus.

The tumor is benign, can be easily removed, and hysterectomy may be required if the entire lesion is not excised and causes abnormal bleeding.

Uterine smooth muscle tumors

Leiomyosarcoma (LMS)

Definition

A malignant neoplasm composed of cells demonstrating smooth muscle differentiation.

Leiomyosarcoma represents a pure uterine sarcoma, comprising slightly over 1% of all uterine malignancies. Its incidence is reported to be 0.3-0.4 per 100 000 women per year (52).

Clinical findings

It is exclusively seen in adults, the median age being 50-55 years. The risk factors which are associated with endometrial carcinoma (such as nulliparity, obesity, hypertension, diabetes mellitus etc.) are not known to be associated with LMS. 52. However, a racial difference is seen in the incidence of LMS, with African American women at a greater risk of developing the disease. The other potential risk factors include oral contraceptive use and tamoxifen 53, 54.

Uterine leiomyosarcoma is rare and in our experience, only 23 leiomyosarcoma (16.2%) were encountered among 142 sarcomatous tumors of uterus (Table 1). Many leiomyomas show prominent nuclear pleomorphism and may be over diagnosed as leiomyosarcoma. Conventionally, a diagnosis of leiomyosarcoma is made only when 2 out of 3 criteria, namely coagulative tumor cell necrosis (CTCN), diffuse significant cytological atypia, and mitotic index (>10 per10 HPF) are met.

Prognosis

LMSs are aggressive tumors, and have tendency to recur locally and / or metastasize; the latter most commonly to lung and liver. Five year overall survival is between 45-65% and the stage is a significant prognostic factor 55.

Smooth Muscle Tumor of Uncertain Malignant Potential (STUMP)

Uterine smooth muscle tumors of uncertain malignant potential (STUMP) are relatively uncommon. They are often unclassifiable by current criteria as unequivocally benign or unequivocally malignant.

The seminal work on problematic uterine smooth muscle neoplasms comes from Bell et al 56 and Phillip et al 56a, and this forms the basis of establishing the diagnostic criteria for accurate interpretation. The issue is to evaluate whether any particular morphological finding is able to reliably predict the biological behavior of the tumor. The various parameters: such as cellularity, mitotic index, degree and extent of atypia, types of necrosis, tumor uterine interface and intravascular growth were extensively studied in 213 patients 56. Out of three univariate predictors, atypia, mitotic index, and coagulative tumor cell necrosis (CTCN), it was concluded that CTCN comes out as the best separating feature between benign and malignant smooth muscle tumors.

Bell et al subdivided STUMP tumors into the following groups:
a) Atypical leiomyoma with low risk of recurrence – diffuse moderate to severe atypia, <10MFs/10hpf and no CTCN
b) Atypical leiomyoma but limited experience

focal moderate to severe atypia, ,20 MFs/10hpf, no CTCN
c) Smooth muscle tumor of low malignant potential
has CTCN, ,mitoses less than 10 MFs/10hpf,absent to mild nuclear atypia

Perhaps the most critical diagnostic issue is to define what constitutes CTCN. Bell et al described it as an abrupt transition from viable cells to necrotic cells without an intervening zone of granulation or hyalinized tissue. Often, there is preservation of the cells in the perivascular location. Hyaline type necrosis, on the other hand, shows a band of paucicellular hyaline collagen seen in between viable and non-viable cells. There is uniform pale outline of tissue including blood vessels. (Figure16).

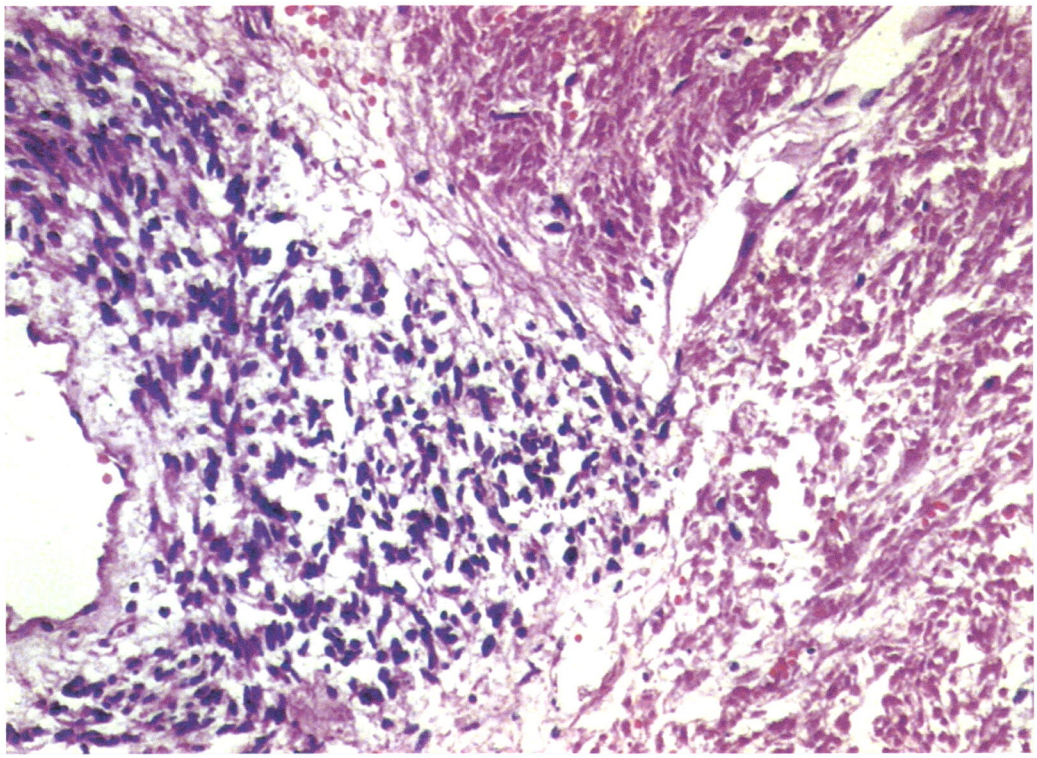

Fig 16: Concentrically arranged perivascular sarcoma cells adjacent to sharply defined zone of coagulative tumor cell necrosis

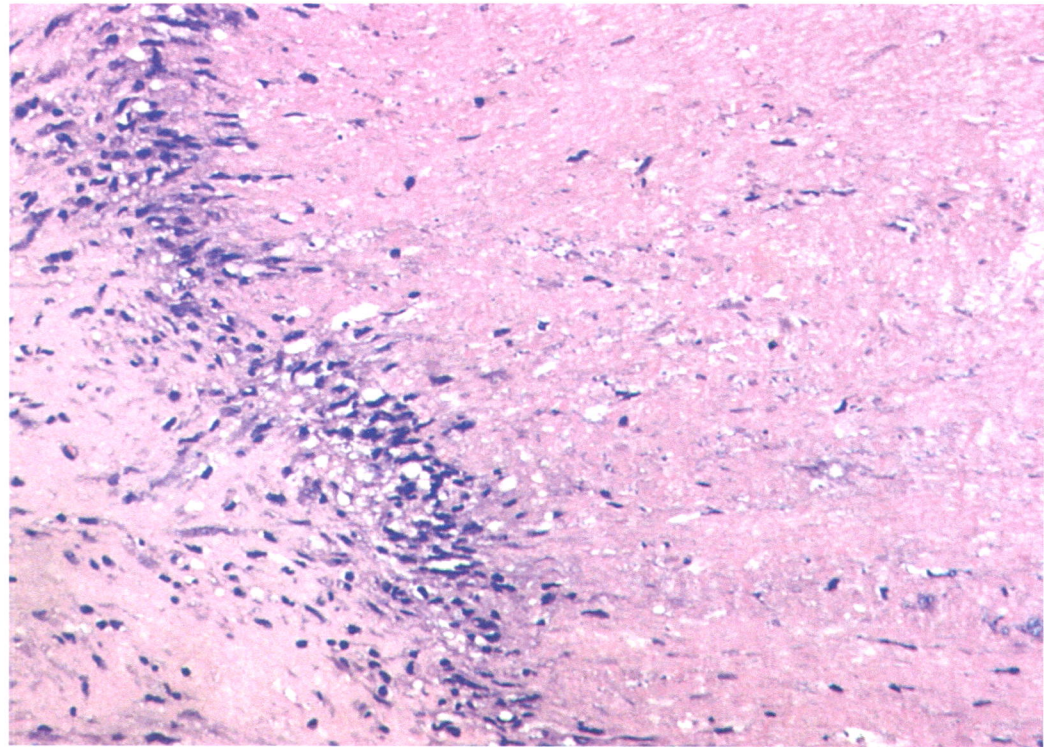

Fig 17.:
Hyaline necrosis
The overall pattern of hyaline necrosis suggested previous infarction with 'walling off' or reparative fibrosis

The third and less common type of necrosis is designated as ulcerative necrosis. This is typically found in submucosal smooth muscle tumors and is associated with inflammatory reaction on the surface. Early phase of hyaline necrosis may not show collagen deposition (Figure 17). We then found preservation of blood vessels and peritheliomatous intact tumor cells in CTCN a reliable point in their distinction.

It should be noted that all the above diagnostic criteria apply to uterine smooth muscle tumors of usual spindle cell differentiation and not applicable to epithelioid and myxoid varieties. If the tumor is predominantly epithelioid, immunohistochemistry is required to prove the cell of origin and to exclude other possibilities such as endometrial stromal sarcoma, pecoma etc.

In our opinion, it is sometimes challenging to distinguish between hyaline necrosis and CTCN, accurately interpret mitotic Figures or decide whether the given tumor is of usual spindle cell variety or epithelioid variety. Alternative interpretation may lead to different diagnostic categories and then it is reasonable to call the lesion as 'smooth muscle tumor of uncertain malignant potential'.

Atypical leiomyoma

(Synonyms: symplastic leiomyoma, bizarre leiomyoma, pleomorphic leiomyoma)

This variant of smooth muscle tumor is characterized by presence of cells with enlarged, coarsely hyperchromatic pleomorphic nuclei. Bizarre nuclear giant cells are often encountered and the nuclei are often smudgy (Figure 18 A). The atypia may be unifocal, multifocal or diffuse. These pleomorphic nuclei may show nuclear pseudo inclusions, multiple nucleated cells, hyperchromasia and abundant eosinophilic cytoplasm. (Figure 18 b) They typically occur in the reproductive age group, with mean age of 40 yrs. 55. According to Downes and Hart 57 the mitotic count may be seen up to 7 per HPF, particularly with tumors having diffuse nuclear atypia. The long term study of patients having tumor with highly bizarre nuclear features have shown a benign biological course.

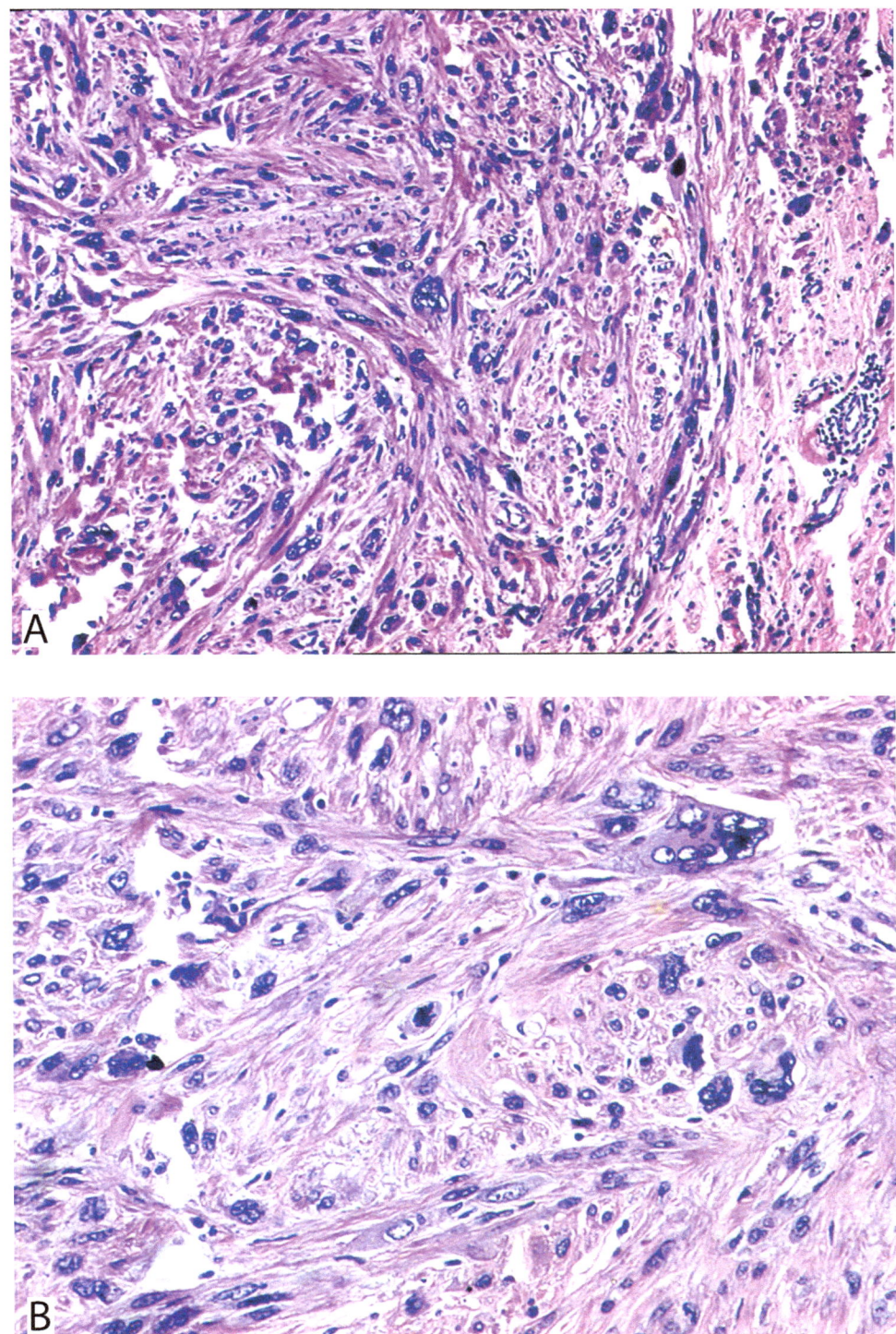

Figure 18 (A) Atypical leiomyoma showing diffuse moderate to severe atypia; (B) note multinucleated tumor giant cells and an atypical mitotic Figure. No coagulative tumor cell necrosis was present in this tumor.

Epithelioid Smooth Muscle Tumors

Smooth muscle cell tumors with epithelioid cell morphology can be benign or malignant and distinction between the two is not always easy. Histologically, epithelioid smooth muscle tumors show contiguous cellular sheets of medium sized round or slightly elongated cells containing acidophilic or clear cytoplasm and enlarged nuclei with inconspicuous nucleoli. The cells express desmin and smooth muscle actin (Figure 19 A, B). A detailed clinicopathologic study of 18 patients with these tumors 58 and literature survey revealed that uterine smooth muscle tumors with predominance of epithelioid cells are extremely uncommon and metastases are infrequent in the malignant counterpart of epithelioid leiomyoma. No single histological feature is predictive of metastatic potential, although epithelioid leiomyosarcoma usually shows significant nuclear atypia, some mitotic activity and tumor necrosis.

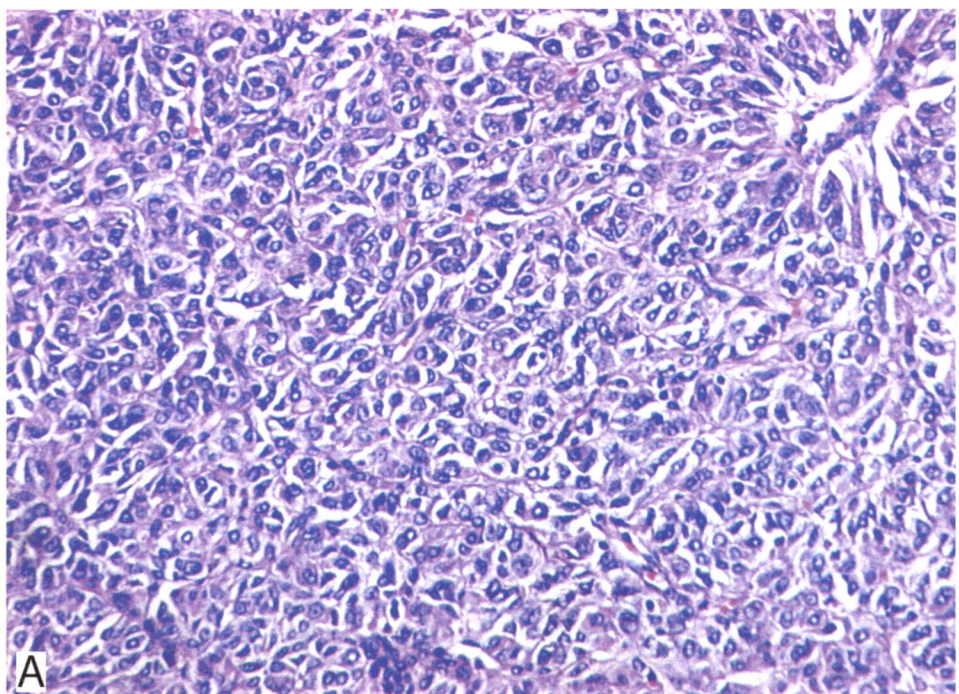

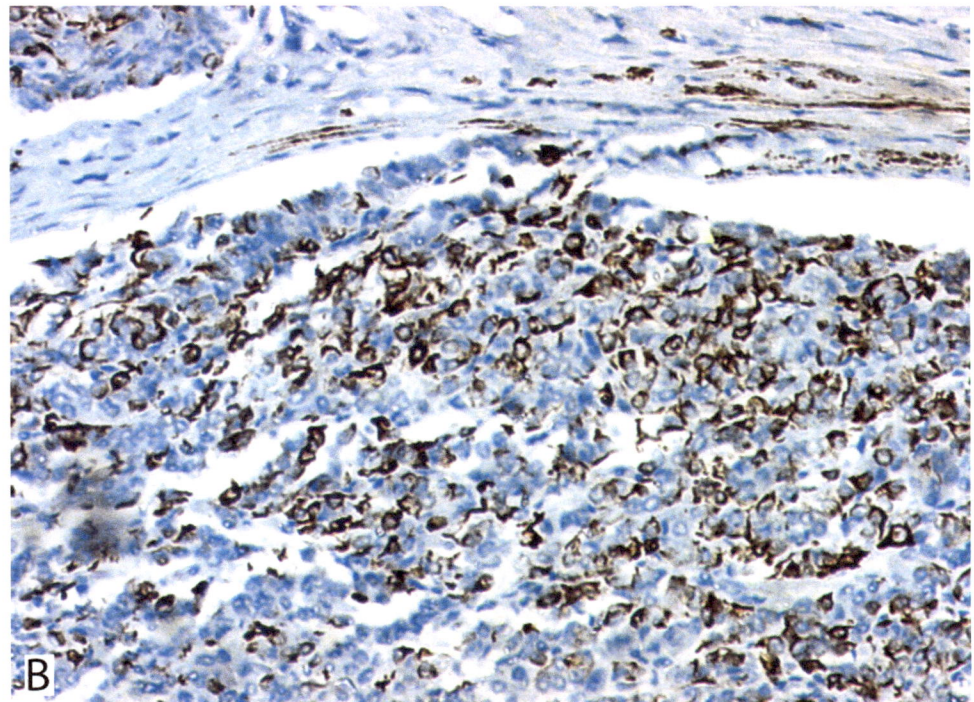

Figure.19 A) Epithelioid smooth muscle tumor; B) desmin positivity

Tumors of the uterine cervix

Table 2 : Tumors of Uterine Cervix (*n*= 2246)** Author's series (1970-2006)	
Adenocarcinoma	128 (5.7%)
Adenoma malignum	2 (0.09%)
Adenoacanthoma	7 (0.31%)
Adenosquamous Carcinoma	14 (0.62%)
Clear cell Carcinoma	8 (0.35%)
Undifferentiated Carcinoma	9 (0.40%)
Carcinoid (neuroendocrine tumor)	3 (0.13%)
Malignant Melanoma	4 (0.18%)
Leiomyosarcoma	2 (0.09%)
Mullerian Adenosarcoma	1 (0.05%)
CIN 3 ***	405 (18%)
(A) Severe Dysplasia	238
(B) CIS	167
Microinvasive Squamous Carcinoma	83 (3.7%)
Invasive Squamous Carcinoma	1580 (70.3%)

** In a total of 6414 cervical biopsies, 2246 (35%) biopsies were of malignant tumors.
*** Severe dysplasia and CIS are considered as synonymous and come under the designation CIN3

Table 3: Tumors of Vagina (*n* = 200) ** Author's series(1970-2006)	
Adenocarcinoma	25 (12.5%)
Metastatic adenocarcinoma (endometrial or cervical primary)	5
Clear cell carcinoma	1
Serous adenocarcinoma	3
Adenoid cystic carcinoma	2
Endodermal sinus tumor	3
Malignant melanoma	7
Malignant mixed Mullerian tumor	3
Rhabdomyosarcoma(4 embryonal and 2 pleomorphic)	6
Sarcoma (NOS)	0
Squamous cell carcinoma	145 (72.5%)

In a total of 698 vaginal biopsies, 200 (28.6%) were accounted for by malignant tumors.

Table 4: Tumors of Vulva (*n* = 70) ** Author's series(1970-2006)	
Squamous Cell Carcinoma	50
CIN 3 (Severe dysplasia + CIS)	4
Microinvasive Squamous Carcinoma	1
Basal Cell Carcinoma	2
Paget's disease (extra mammary)	2
Adenocarcinoma (NOS)	1
Clear Cell Carcinoma	1
Malignant Melanoma	4
Dermatofibroma Protuberance	1
Fibromatosis	1
Rhabdomyosarcoma (pleomorphic)	2
Aggressive *Angiomyxoma* (Recurrent)	1

**In a total of 348 vulval biopsies, 70 (20%) were accounted for by malignant tumors.

Minimal Deviation Adenocarcinoma of Cervix

Definition

Minimal deviation adenocarcinoma (MDA), also known as adenoma malignum, is extremely well differentiated variant of cervical adenocarcinoma, accounting for 1% to 3% of all cervical adenocarcinomas. Silverberg and Hunt introduced the term "minimal deviation adenocarcinoma" for this lesion because of its close resemblance to normal endocervical glands 59.

Clinical findings

In a review of 389 primary adenocarcinomas of the cervix on files of AFIP, only 1%-3% cases represented MDA 60. Patients age ranged from 25 to 72 years with average of 42 years. MDAs are usually found to be negative for HPV 61. Minimal deviation adenocarcinomas of cervix and ovarian sex cord tumor with annular tubules have been found to be strongly associated with Peutz-Jeghers syndrome 62. MDAs are frequently associated with a profuse watery, mucinous discharge or abnormal vaginal bleeding.

Gross

On colposcopy, cervix with early stage of MDA can appear normal and in advanced stage polypoid lesion or irregularities of the cervix will be seen.

Microscopic

The MDA is histologically characterized by cytologically low grade but architecturally atypical glands that vary in size, shape and arrangement. Features that are most helpful in distinguishing MDA from benign endocervical glandular lesions are: the presence of markedly irregular abnormally shaped glands, invasion in the cervical stroma, loose edematous or desmoplastic stromal response (Figure 20 A-E), foci of glands with significant atypia, and perineural invasion. The latter two microscopic features are not always found to be present. Thus, MDA appears deceptively benign and must be differentiated from benign endocervical glandular proliferative lesions. MDA usually involves more than 2/3rds thickness of cervical wall and should be regarded as invasive because the normal endocervical crypts do not extend beyond 7 mm 63

Because the depth of penetration of the glands is an essential histological feature of MDA in most cases, the diagnosis cannot be made on a routine cervical biopsy; either a cone biopsy or hysterectomy specimen will be required to arrive at a diagnosis.

Immunohistochemistry

Cytoplasmic staining of tumor cells for carcinoembryonic antigen (CEA) is a very reliable diagnostic criterion, and effectively separates benign endocervical proliferations from MDA (Figure 20 F, G).Ki 67 proliferation index is high in this bland and benign appearing tumor 64

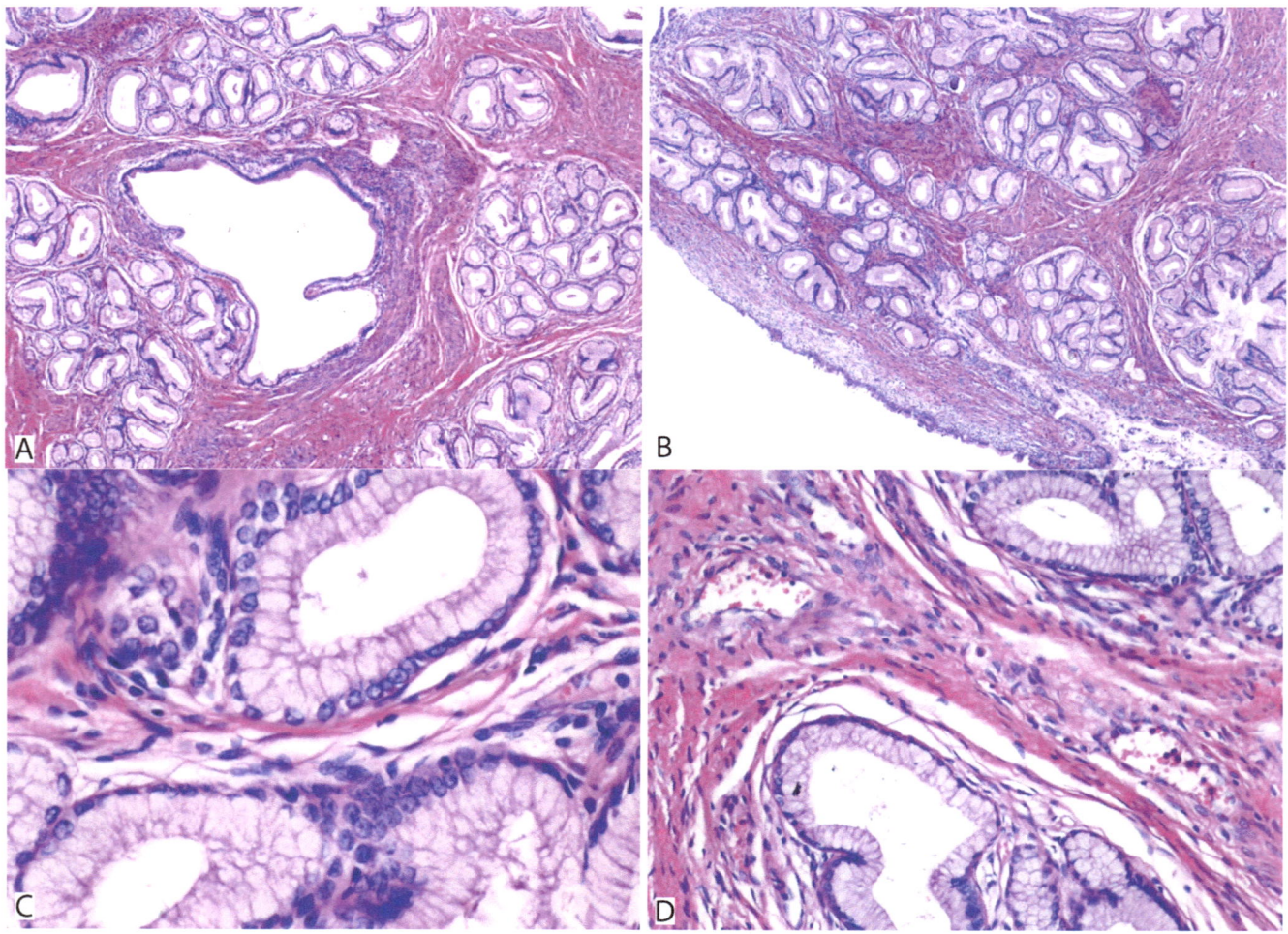

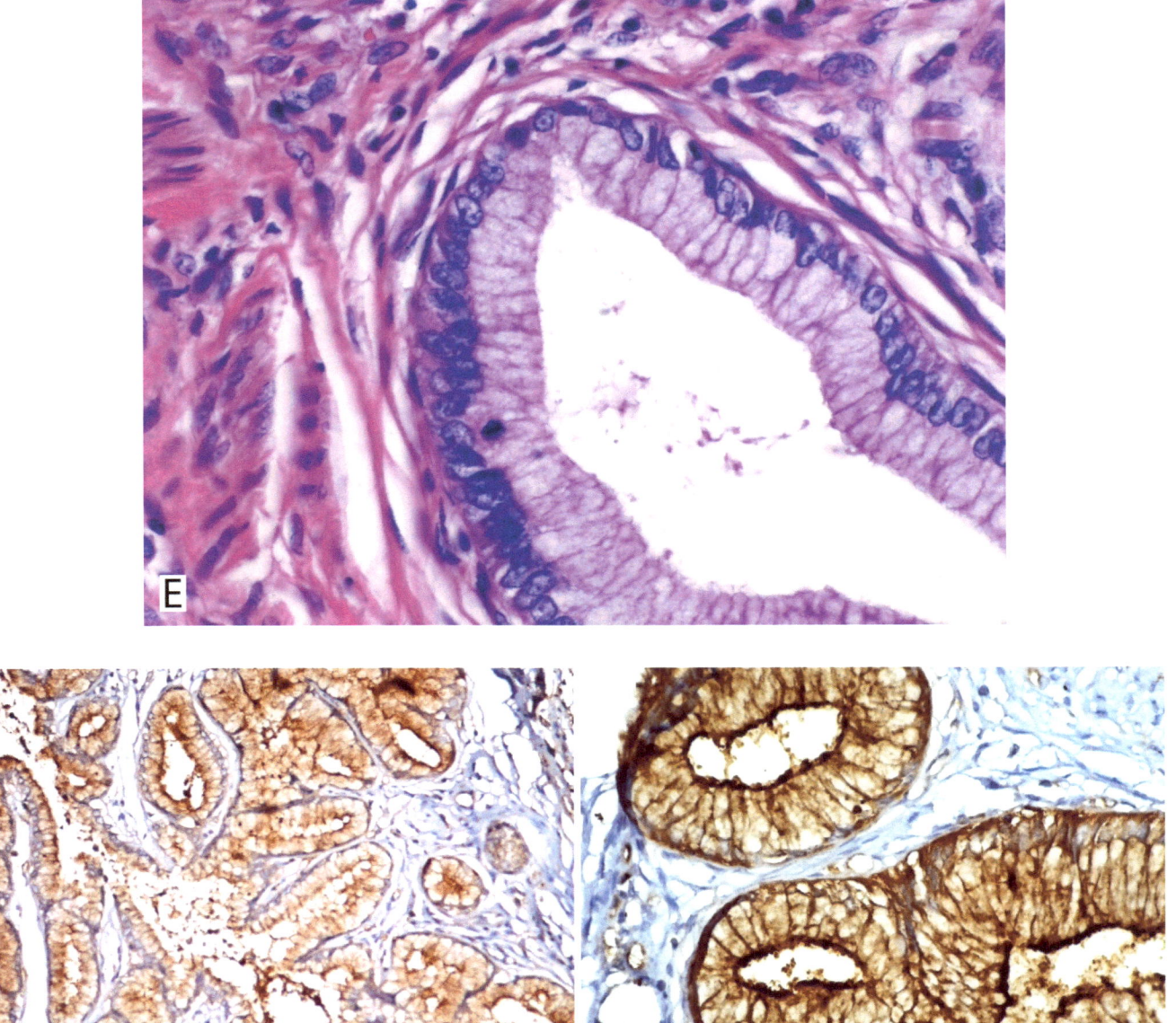

Figure 20 (A,B) large lobules of loosely arranged disoriented endocervical glands situated deep in the cervical stroma; (C,D) medium power view of the endocervical neoplastic glands; E- high power view shows lack of significant anaplasia, note small nucleoli; (F,G) CEA is expressed in membrane and cytoplasm of the neoplastic glands

Prognosis

Despite radical therapy in most of the cases, the prognosis is poor. Follow up data in 22 of 26 cases revealed that 13 died of recurrent of tumor, 4 were alive with disease and only 3 were disease free for 2 year or more 64.

Glandular Lesions of Cervix Mimicking Adenocarcinoma

Neoplastic and presumed preneoplastic endocervical glandular lesions are increasingly being reported in the literature. In developed countries, organized cervical screening programs have led to a decrease in incidence of invasive squamous carcinoma and relative increase in the incidence of endocervical adenocarcinoma. There is a better awareness on the part of surgical pathologists with a focus on precursors and possible precursor lesions of endocervical adenocarcinoma. Some of the benign mimics of cervical adenocarcinoma that pose a diagnostic problem are discussed here, along with the discussion on cervical glandular intraepithelial neoplasia 65, 66, 67.

Many types of endocervical glandular proliferations have been described and some of these conditions will be described.

Deep cervical glands and cysts:

Some endocervical crypts, especially when dilated, are present deep within the cervical stroma and may be confused with minimal deviation adenocarcinoma. However, these do not exhibit irregular stromal infiltration and there is no stromal response.

Tuboendometrioid Metaplasia (TEM) and Endometriosis

TEM, in the experience of the experts, is the most common lesion, to be misdiagnosed as cervical glandular intraepithelial neoplasia (CGIN). It may occur de novo, but is especially common following diathermy cone or a LEEP procedure. It probably represents aberrant differentiation or metaplasia following injury. TEM is characterized by replacement of normal endocervical glands by hyperchromatic, closely packed cuboidal to columnar cells with high N/C ratio (Figure 21 A, B). The best clue to diagnosis is the presence of cilia on the luminal border of some of the cells (Figure 21 C). If need be, immunohistochemical staining for MIB-1 ,bcl-2 and P16 should be carried out. High grade CGIN will show high MIB-1 index, negative bcl-2 staining and diffuse positivity for P16 67, 68, 69, 70,71

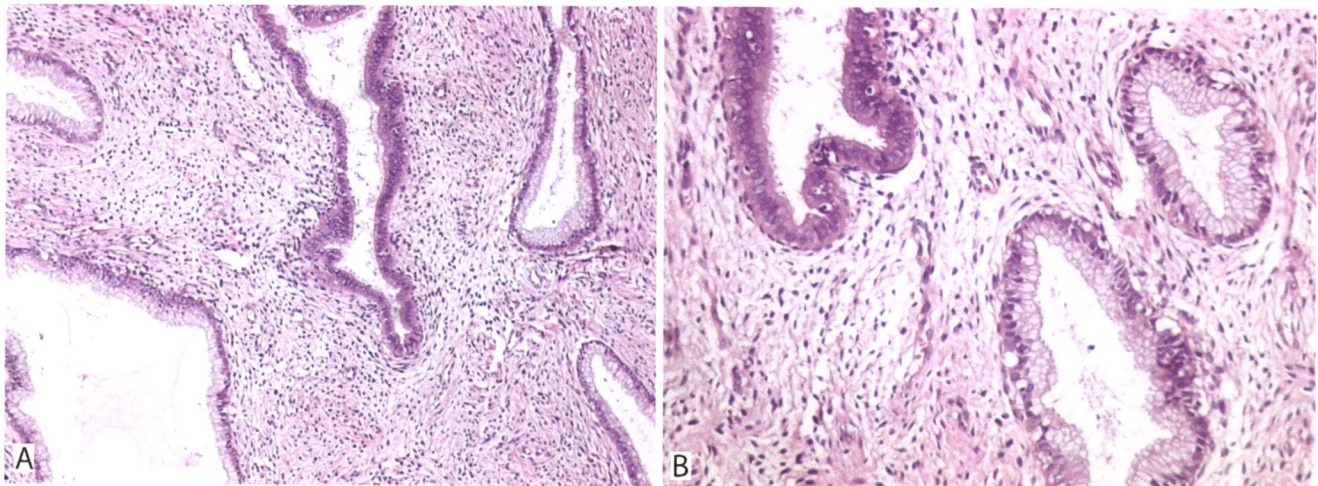

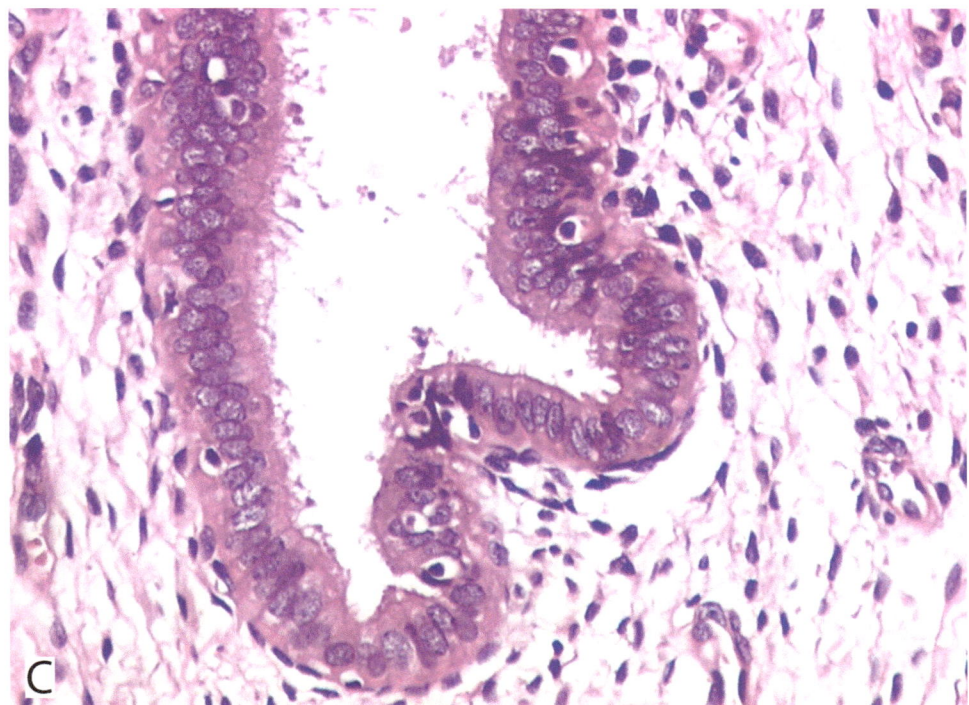

Figure 21 Tubo-endometrioid metaplasia :(A) scanner view of normal endocervical glands with one dark staining metaplastic gland; (B) medium power view ; (C) high power view of the gland with endometrioid metaplasia: Note enlarged hyperchromatic nuclei and presence of cilia

Microglandular Adenosis (MGA) or hyperplasia

It is a common lesion, thought to be a result of progesterone influence of pregnancy, but it is not necessarily so. Microscopically, MGA is characterized by presence of closely packed small glands lined by regular cuboidal epithelial cells with vesicular nuclei. Mitotic Figures are uncommon, but may be found. Often seen are supra or infranuclear vacuolations, neutrophils infiltrating the cells and chronic inflammation especially plasma cells in the stroma. Reserve cell hyperplasia, immature squamous metaplasia are also seen (Figure 22 A-D). The atypical features include, edema, stromal hyalinization and signet ring cells. It is these changes which can lead to confusion with clear cell adenocarcinoma or cervical glandular intraepithelial neoplasia (CGIN), but the latter two generally have higher mitotic rate than MGA. Atypical mitoses are often seen and nuclei are not vesicular. In difficult cases, immunohistochemistry with CEA is suggested. Diffuse cytoplasmic positivity with CEA is generally seen in neoplasia, and favors a diagnosis of adenocarcinoma 65. In difficult cases, it is helpful to carry out Ki 67 immunostaining, which usually shows low grade proliferation index (Figure 22 E, F).72

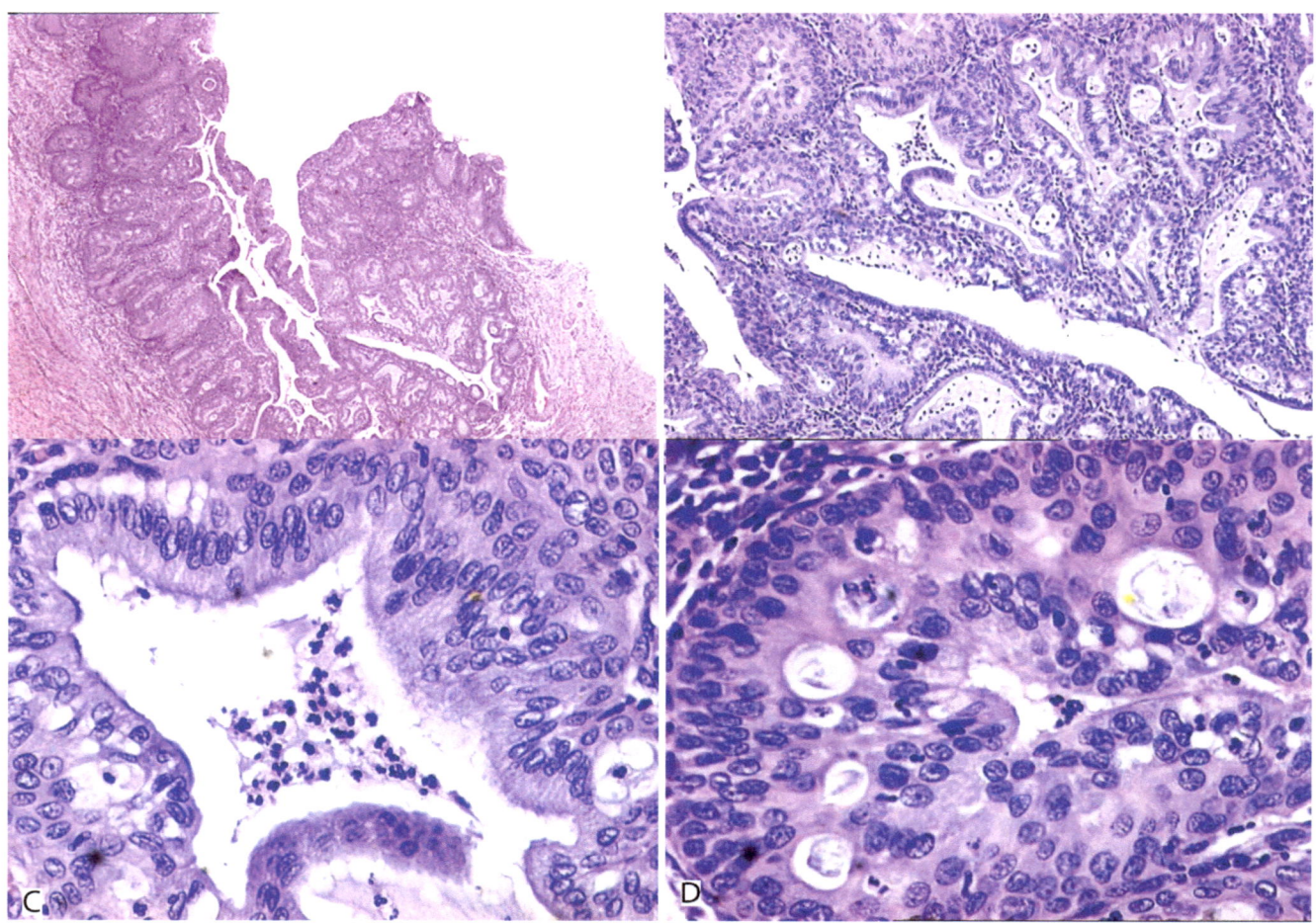

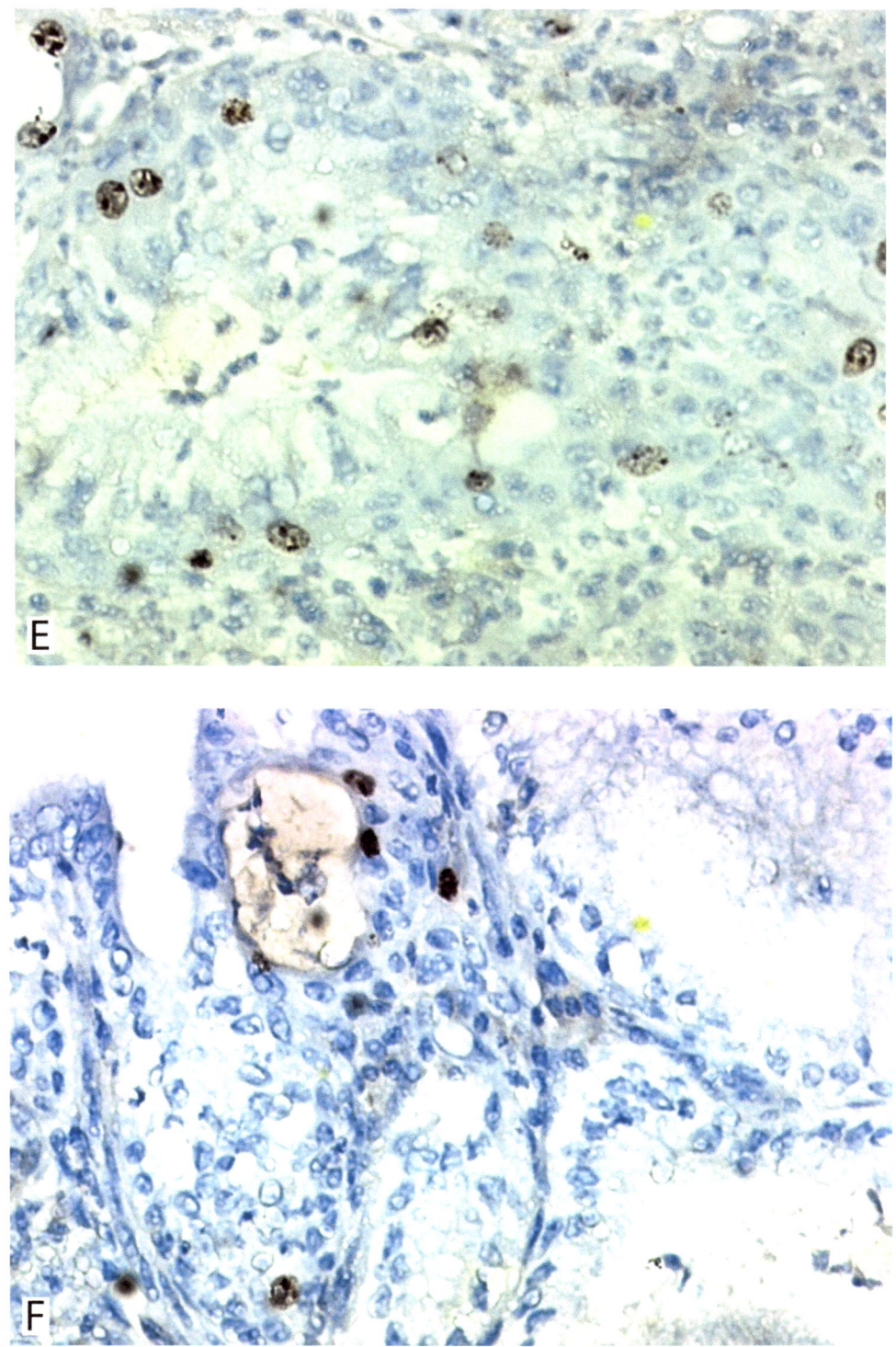

Figure 22 Micro glandular hyperplasia: (A, B) low power view; (C, D) high power view; (E, F) Low Ki 67 proliferation index

Mesonephric remnants

These are the vestigial elements of the distal ends of the mesonephric ducts, and can be found in 1% to 22% of the adult cervices. The variability in reporting its occurrence is largely dependent on how extensively the cervix is sampled. Mesonephric remnants are most commonly present in the lateral aspect of the cervix, and show small tubules, lined by non-ciliated low cuboidal epithelium. Some tubules typically contain eosinophilic luminal secretions (Figure 23 A-D).73

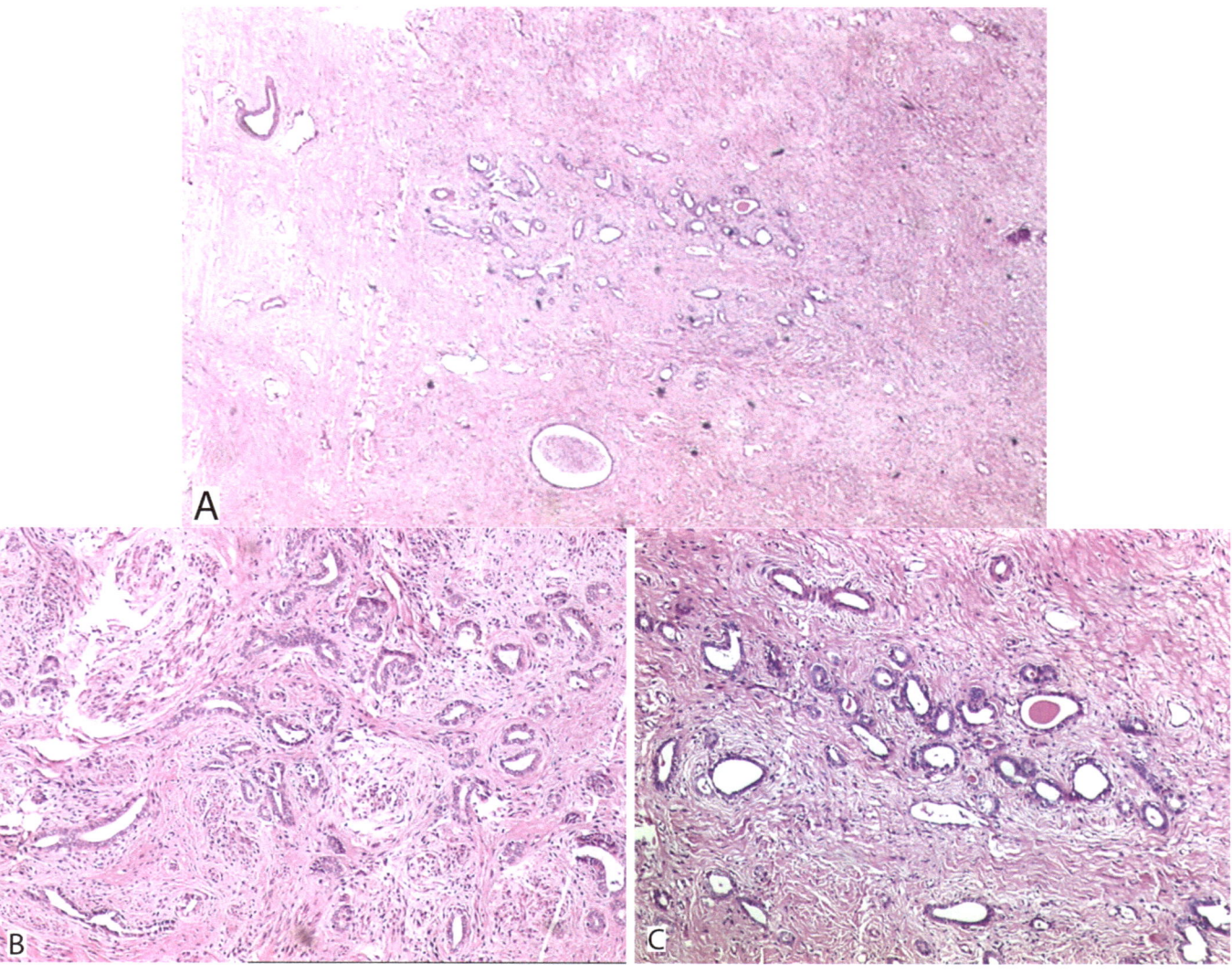

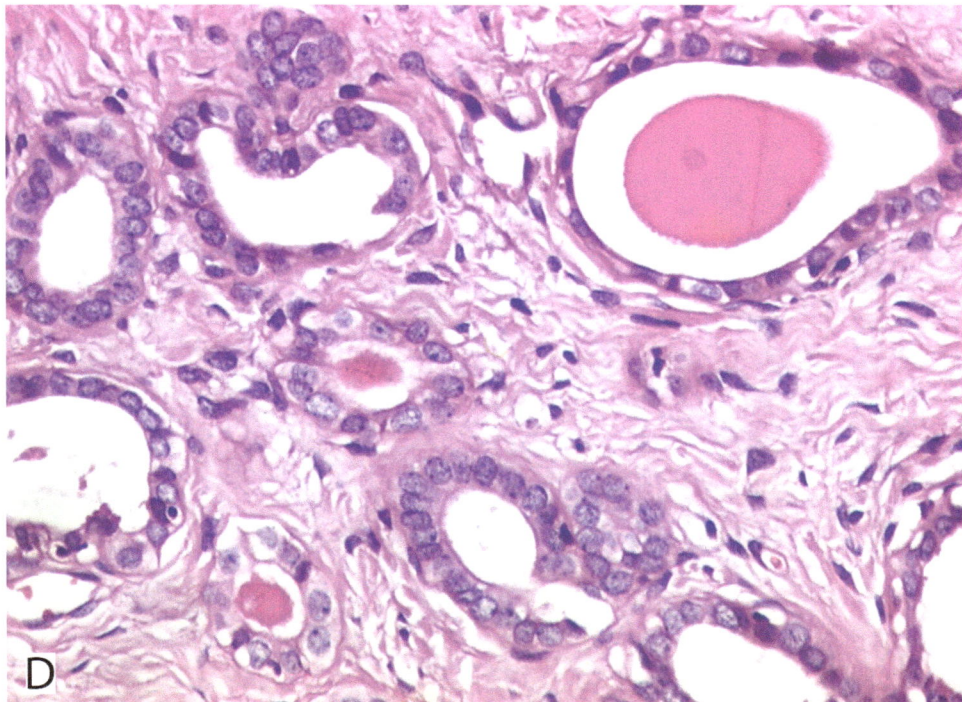

Figure 23 Mesonephric remnants: (A) Scanner view of loose clusters of tubules located deep in the cervical wall; (B & C) more details of above Figure; (D) High power view-tubules lined by non-ciliated cuboidal cells, eosinophilic material in the lumina

Endocervical Glandular Dysplasia

Definition

A glandular lesion characterized by significant nuclear abnormalities that are more striking than those in glandular atypia but fall short of the criteria for adenocarcinoma

The terminology of Cervical Glandular Intraepithelial Neoplasia (CGIN) is being used and a two tier grading system of low grade CGIN and high grade CGIN is recommended.

Morphological features of cervical Glandular Intraepithelial Neoplasia (CGIN)

A combination of cytological and architectural features is usually present. Cytological features include nuclear stratification, pleomorphism, overlapping. Nucleoli, loss of polarity and apoptotic bodies are seen in high grade CGIN. Architectural features (all of which may not be present), include crowding , branching, budding, intraluminal papillary projections and cribriforming. There is often an abrupt transition within an individual crypt between normal endocervical crypt and CGIN (Figure 24A, B). High grade CGIN is a relatively robust diagnosis amongst the histopathologists, although its distinction from early invasive adenocarcinoma can be extremely difficult (Figure 24 C-E). The recognition of low grade CGIN is more problematic and can be under diagnosed. CGIN may be associated with intraepithelial squamous lesion. 74,75

The entity of early invasive or microinvasive adenocarcinoma is controversial. There are also practical problems in identifying microinvasive adenocarcinoma. Nevertheless it is recommended that FIGO classification be adopted.

Treatment Implications

Previously, management of high grade CGIN was usually by hysterectomy. Recently there has been a tendency to treat high grade CGIN with cone biopsy or LEEP, especially in young women who wish to retain their fertility. For conservative treatment, cytological follow up is required. Treatment of low grade CGIN is generally similar to that of high grade CGIN. Pathologists feel that a diagnosis of low grade CGIN is not robust and thus hysterectomy for a diagnosis of Low grade CGIN may be an overtreatment. Hence, the diagnosis of low grade CGIN should be made with great care.

TUMORS OF THE UTERINE CERVIX

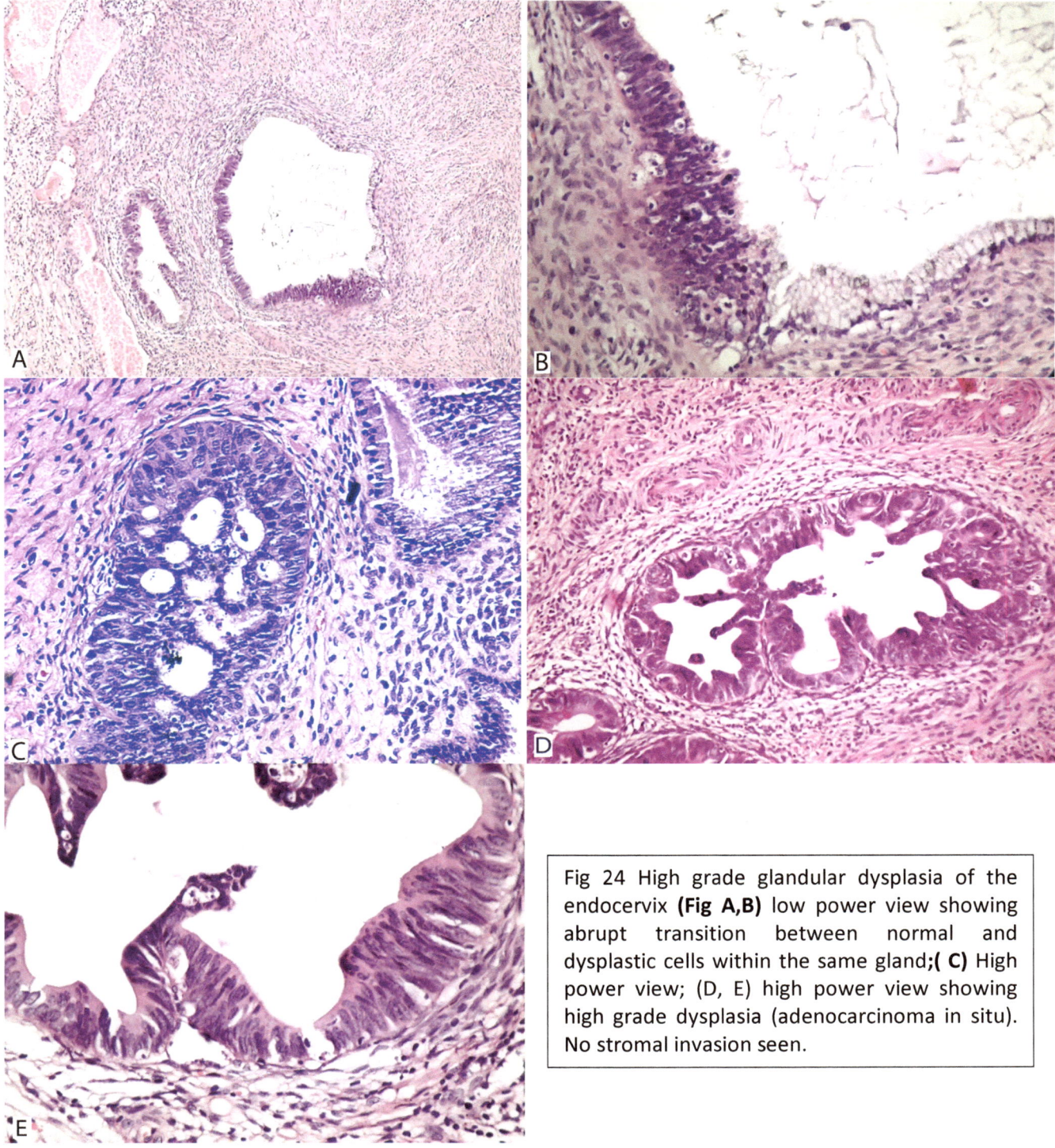

Fig 24 High grade glandular dysplasia of the endocervix **(Fig A,B)** low power view showing abrupt transition between normal and dysplastic cells within the same gland;**(C)** High power view; (D, E) high power view showing high grade dysplasia (adenocarcinoma in situ). No stromal invasion seen.

Malignant Melanoma of Female Genital Tract

Mucosal Melanoma

Mucosal melanoma is a rare cancer that is clearly distinct from its cutaneous counterpart in biological, clinical course and prognosis. Melanomas of head and neck, the female genital tract and the ano-rectum are three most common sites of mucosal melanoma. Melanomas of head and neck region are discussed in detail in Chapter 1 on Head & Neck.

Primary mucosal melanomas of the female genital tract account for 18% of all mucosal melanomas 76. One large retrospective study of 2882 patients with melanoma reported that 50 (1.8%) patients had amelanotic melanoma 77. If the possibility of amelanotic melanoma is not thought of, the tumor can be easily misdiagnosed as a carcinoma, sarcoma or lymphoma. However, this difficulty is easily solved by application of immunohistochemical markers for melanocytes, namely; S100, HMB 45, and Melan A, which have vastly improved the diagnostic accuracy of amelanotic melanoma 78. Demonstration of melanosomes and pre melanosomes on electron microscopy is the most authentic method of diagnosis of amelanotic melanoma.

Of the mucosal melanomas among female genital tract, 76.7% are vulvar, 19.8% vaginal and cervical least common. The rate for mucosal melanoma per million per year is 2.2 compared to 153.5 for cutaneous melanoma 79, 76.

There are important differences between cutaneous melanoma and mucosal melanoma. Amelanotic melanoma occurs in 1.8% to 8.1% of cutaneous melanoma and in 20% to 25% in mucosal melanoma. Activating mutations in the c-KIT gene are detected in some cases of malignant melanoma: <5% in cutaneous melanoma and 15%-22% in mucosal melanoma. These issues have obvious therapeutic and prognostic implications 80.

Vulvar Melanoma

Melanoma is the second most common vulvar malignancy, after squamous cell carcinoma in our series, there were 59 cases of squamous carcinoma and 4 cases melanoma. Symptoms at the presentation are similar to those of other gynecological tumors and include: bleeding, discharge, pruritus, burning pain, dysuria and the presence of a polypoid mass or ulceration. Most of these lesions are black or grey-black in color and some are amelanotic. Most melanomas arising from labia majora area considered cutaneous, whereas those arising from labia minor are considered to be mucosal in origin 81.The age of occurrence in large series varied from 58-79 years and all women were postmenopausal.

Prognosis of melanoma.

In the Swedish study, the 5 year rate was 35%, with rates of 26.8% and 65.2% for node-positive and node-negative vulvar melanomas, respectively. The observed and relative survival rates at 10 years were 23% and 44% respectively 81. In cases of recurrent melanomas the 5 year survival rate is a mere 5% 82.

Paget's disease of Vulva

This disease is being discussed and illustrated here because of its close histological resemblance to superficial spreading melanoma. Paget's disease of vulva presents as either erythematous or an eczematous lesion that appears as red to pink areas with white islands of hyperkeratosis. The lesion can be focal or involves perianal region and medial aspects of upper thigh. The affected women are postmenopausal with median age of 70 years and more than half complain of pruritus. There is a primary cutaneous Paget's disease in the form of in situ carcinoma in epidermis or similar lesion with invasion or a manifestation of underlying cutaneous neoplasm. And there is secondary Paget's disease with an adjacent ano-rectal or urothelial intraepithelial carcinoma 83, 84.

Paget's cells are large with abundant cytoplasm, large nuclei and prominent nucleoli and they are situated within the epidermis. Paget's cells have granular or vacuolated cytoplasm and keratinocytes possess solid acidophilic cytoplasm, the distinction between two cells types is easy. The Paget's cells lie in singles or small groups within the base of epidermis and may populate ("Pagetoid spread") the upper reaches of the epidermis (Figure 25 A, B).

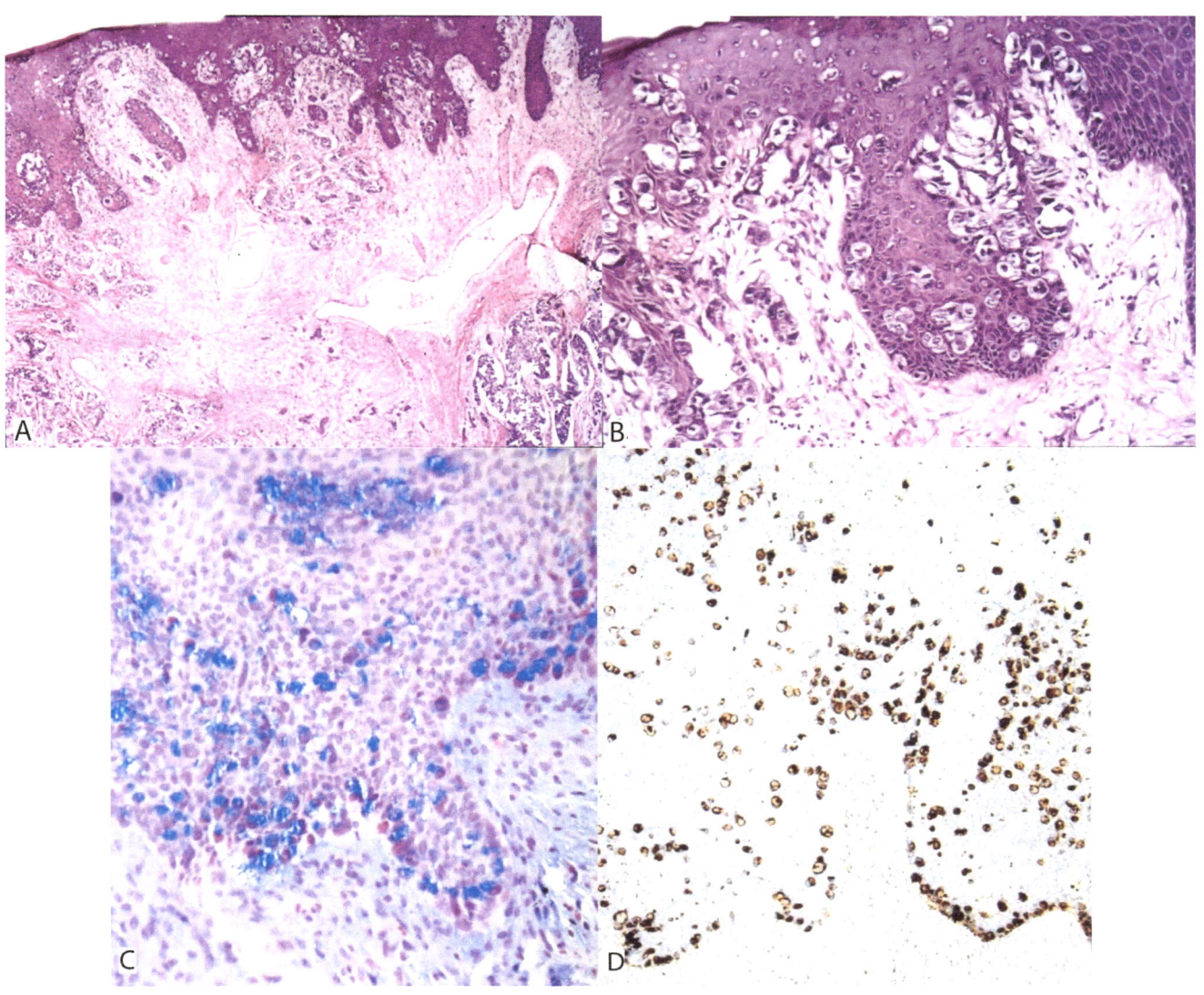

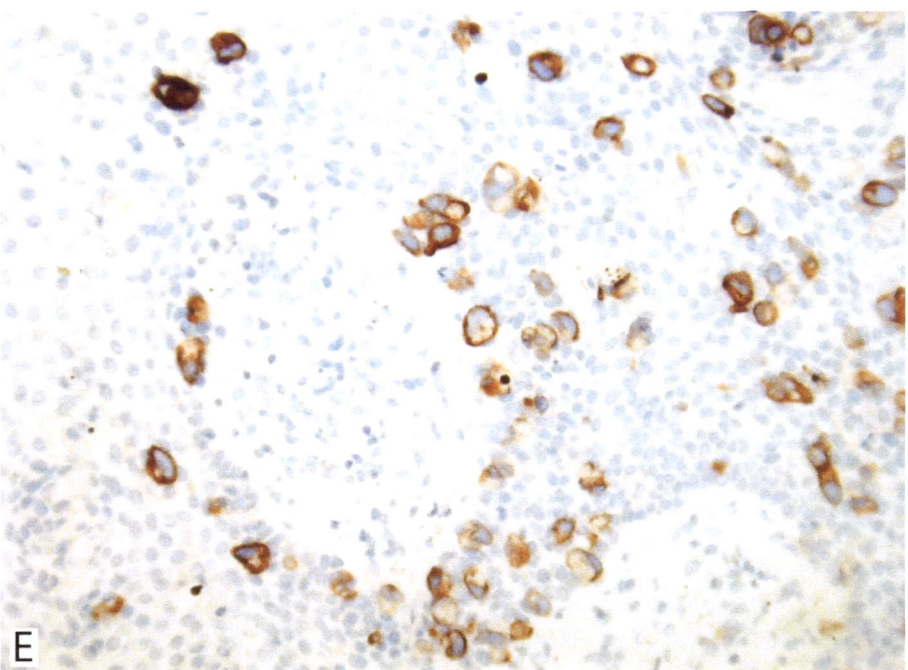

Figure 25 Extra mammary Paget's disease of vulva: (A, B) acanthotic epidermis with large carcinoma cells in the suprabasal region; (C) Alcian Blue and PAS stain; (D) CEA expressed by the tumor cells; (E) CK7 expressed in the cytoplasm.

Differential Diagnosis

The histological features described above can also be seen in cases of superficial spreading melanoma, VIN, and dysplastic nevus. Immunohistochemical study offers great help to particularly differentiate superficial spreading melanoma from Paget's disease., a disease which has low morbidity and mortality, Melanoma markers: HMB 45, S100 and Melan A are readily expressed by melanoma cells and Paget's cells are specifically stained with Alcian blue-PAS, CEA and CK 7 (Figure 25 C-E) 85, 86.

Vaginal Melanoma

The clinical presentation, gross and microscopic findings (described in vulvar melanoma) are almost similar in melanomas of vulva, vagina and cervix and therefore not repeated here.

More than 155 cases of vaginal melanomas have been reported, representing less than 5% of the malignant neoplasms of vagina and less than 1% of all melanomas 87. Among mucosal melanomas, primary melanoma of the vagina is extremely rare, and its very existence was once disputed by some authors. In one autopsy study, melanocytes were identified in the basal layer of the vagina in 3 of 100 women. It has been suggested that such a condition, referred to as benign melanosis, is the setting from which melanoma may arise 88. The presence of melanocytes in the mucosa provides a theoretical cell of origin for malignant melanoma of vagina. Several cases of primary malignant melanoma associated with multifocal melanosis of the vaginal mucosa have been reported. The foci of melanosis occur adjacent to or at a distance from the primary lesion. Almost one-third of malignant melanomas of the oral mucosa among Japanese were found to be associated with pre-existent mucosal melanosis 89.

Prognosis

Malignant vaginal melanoma, even when localized at presentation, has a very poor prognosis. Patients treated surgically have longer survival than those treated non-surgically. Radiotherapy after wide excision reduces local but not the distant recurrences 90. The National Cancer Data Base Report on Cancer of the Vagina revealed that the 5 year survival for a series of 76 vaginal melanoma patients, diagnosed between1985-1989, was only 14%! 91

Cervical Melanoma

Vast majority of melanomas of female genital tract occur in vulva and vagina. Primary melanoma of the uterine cervix is extremely rare, accounting for only 3% to 9% of gynecological melanomas, and it is 5 times less common than primary melanoma of vagina and vulva 92. Only 60 cases of cervical melanoma have been reported as of 2012 93.

Cervical melanoma arises from melanocytic cells of the cervix; in fact the cervical epithelium is capable of forming the complete spectrum of melanocytic lesions, from benign lentiginous to blue nevi to melanoma 19. In most instances, the lesion is pigmented and dark brown to black (Figure 26 A, B), and histologically it is identical to melanoma arising in the skin and extra genital mucous membranes. Rarely cervical malignant melanoma can be composed of clear cells and may show intracytoplasmic melanin granule (Figure 26 C, D).Few tumors are amelanotic and have to be distinguished from undifferentiated carcinoma.

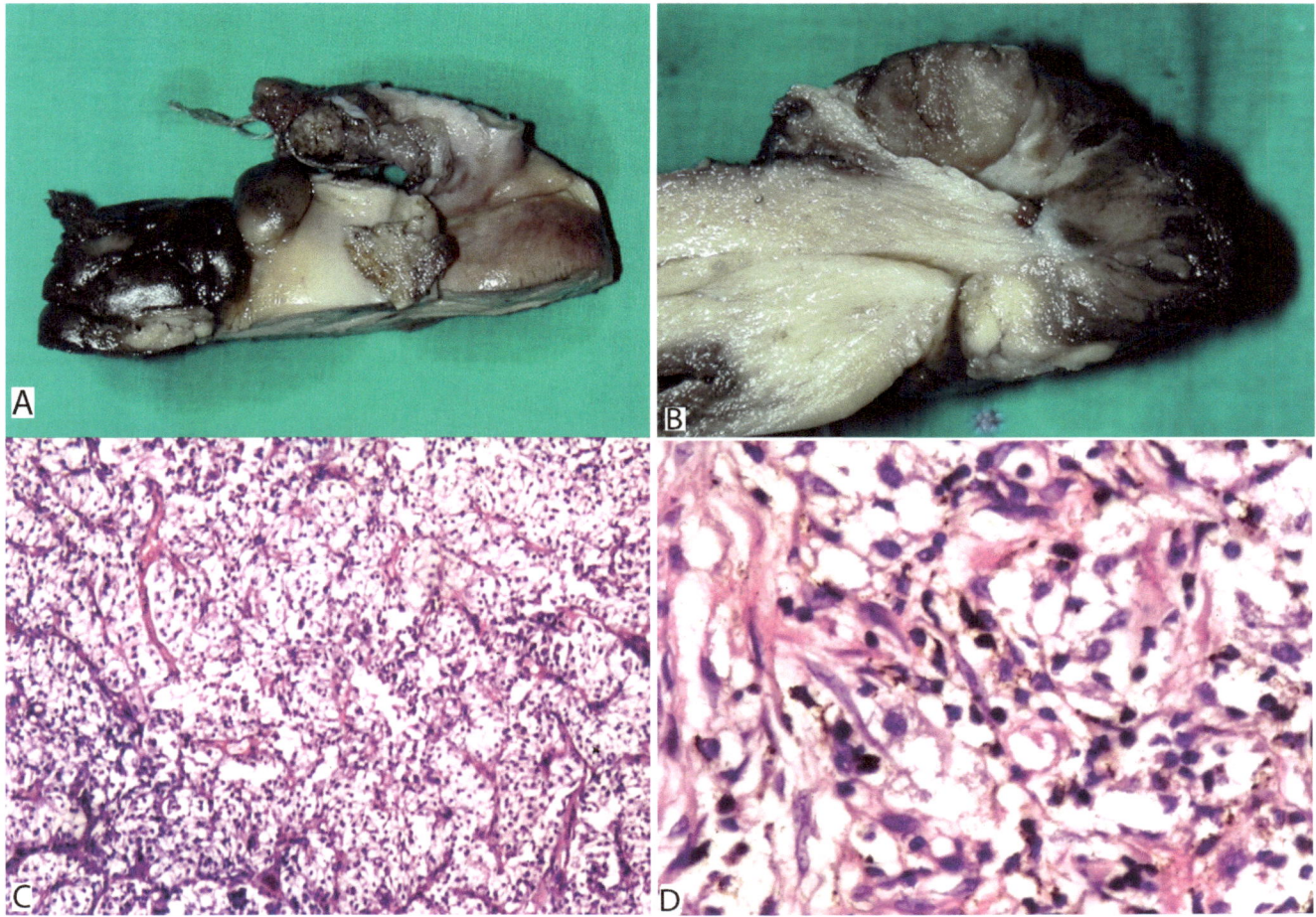

Figure 26 (A, B) Portio cervix shows black discoloration; C- Clear cell morphology of malignant melanoma; D-scattered tumor cells display cytoplasmic course brownish black pigment

Prognosis

The prognosis of primary malignant melanoma of cervix is poor, with 40% 5-year survival for patients with Stage I disease and only 14% 5-year survival rate for patients with high stage disease 94, 95.

Sarcoma Botryoides (Embryonal Rhabdomyosarcoma)

Embryonal rhabdomyosarcoma is the most common malignant tumor of the vagina in infants and children, accounting for 4% to 6% of all malignancies in this age group 96. It also rarely occurs in cervix or uterine fundus. The botryoides subtype of embryonal rhabdomyosarcoma accounts for about 10% of all rhabdomyosarcoma cases and arises under the mucosal surface of body orifices such as the vagina, cervix and urinary bladder 97. Nearly 90% of cases are diagnosed before the age of 5 years and mean age at diagnosis is 2 years. In a 10 year period, 4885 cases of vaginal cancer were submitted to National Cancer Data Base 98, of which vaginal sarcomas accounted for only 135 (2.76%) cases. In this review, 30 sarcomas (22%) were in children under 14 years and 9 were in infants age <1 year.

Gross

It presents as a conglomerate of soft polypoid masses resembling grapes [Greek Botryose: grapes), hence the name. The gross appearance seen in the Figure (Figure 27 A) is quite vivid but is not always present. Sarcoma Botyroides belongs to the group called embryonal rhabdomyosarcoma, which also includes the subtype alveolar rhabdomyosarcoma.

Microscopic

The tumor is characterized by an abundant myxoid stroma containing a small population of undifferentiated round or spindle cells with bright acidophilic cytoplasm suggestive of rhabdomyoblastic differentiation. Cross striations may or may not be present and more often rhabdomyoblastic appearance in the form of strap and tadpole shaped cells is missing. At times, the cell population is so sparse that the malignant nature of the tumor may not be appreciated on a small biopsy, unless the gross clinical appearance is diagnostic. A useful diagnostic feature is the crowding of the tumor cells around blood vessels and formation of distinctive sub epithelial cellular zone, the so-called cambium layer (Figure 27 B, C)

Immunohistochemistry

Desmin (Figure 27 D) and myogenin are expressed in about 96% of cases and proliferative activity, as assessed by Ki-67 expression, is markedly elevated in all these tumors 99.

SARCOMA BOTRYOIDES (EMBRYONAL RHABDOMYOSARCOMA)

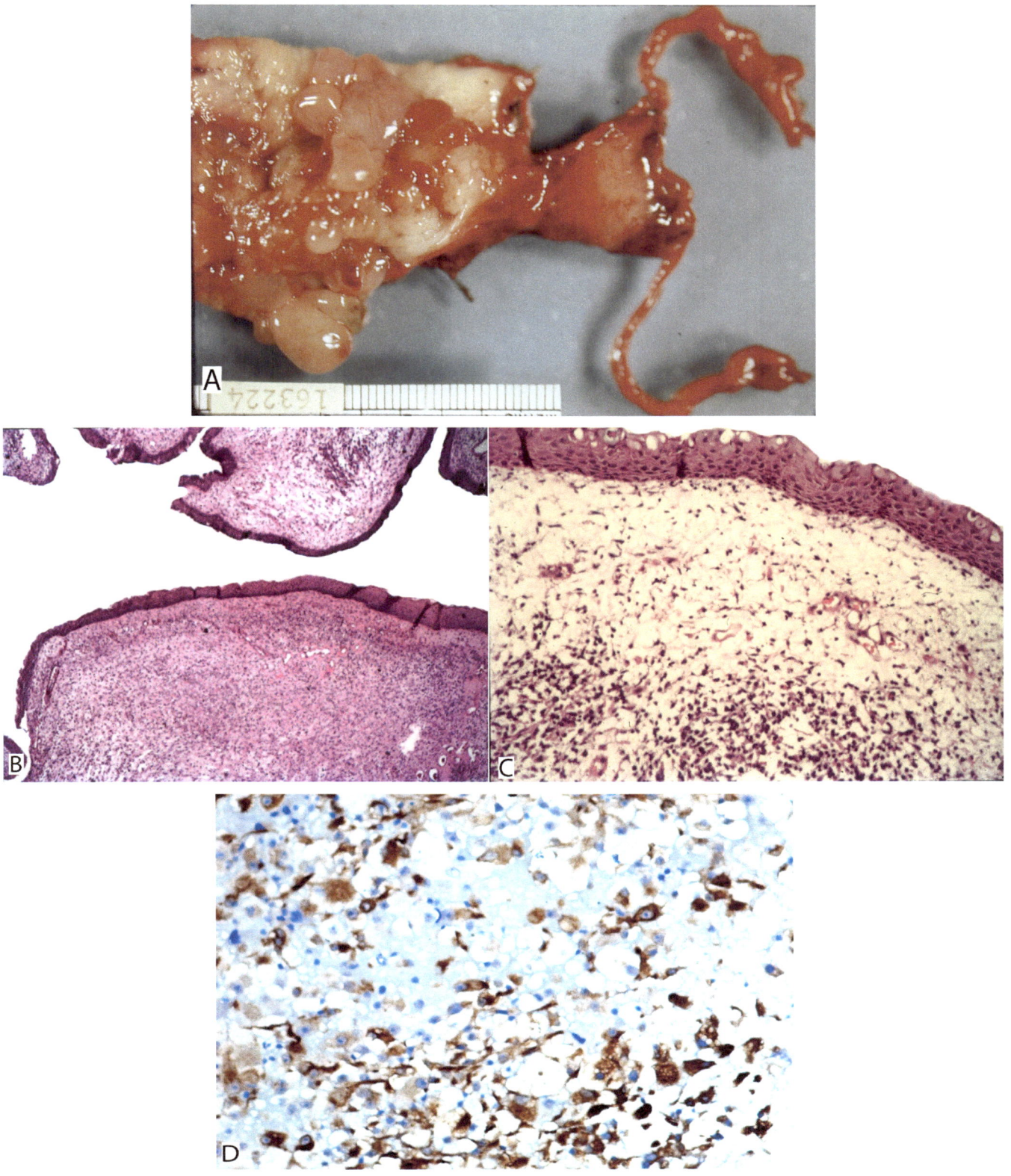

Figure 27 (A) Vagina distended with large growth of slightly translucent 'cystic' nodules; (B) Squamous mucosa overlying edematous paucicellular sarcoma; (C) Condensed tumor cells forming cambium layer in the deeper tissue; D- Strong desmin positivity in the tumor cells

Prognosis

In the M D Anderson hospital experience of 8 cases of alveolar rhabdomyosarcoma in the female genitalia, 5 died within 9 months, 1 died 27 months after diagnosis and only 2 are 5-year survivors 100.

Gestational Trophoblastic diseases

Gestational trophoblastic diseases comprise a heterogeneous group of lesions having specific clinical features, morphological characteristics and variable biological behavior. A number of these lesions are malignant and some show low grade malignant behavior but are curable with appropriate management. Exaggerated placental site lesion and placental site nodules are two clearly benign entities, which are included because these must be histologically distinguished from trophoblastic tumors which may have malignant potential. Recent studies with larger case series have shown profound differences in the morphology and clinical out come and such studies underline the importance of uniform histological classification to facilitate standard reporting of data and to ensure appropriate management. The author's cases of gestational trophoblastic diseases have been presented within the framework of WHO classification. It is noted that we have not seen a case of epithelioid trophoblastic tumor or placental site nodule. The series highlights the rarity of placental site trophoblastic tumor, of which only three cases (0.73%) have been encountered among 412 cases in the group. This entity, a prototype of placental site trophoblastic lesions is being discussed at length.

WHO Classification of Gestational Trophoblastic diseases

Table 5 Gestational Trophoblastic Tumors (n = 397): Author's series (1970-2006),	
Hydatidiform mole (n =349)	
Complete mole	324
Partial mole	25
Invasive mole("chorioadenoma destruens")	9
Trophoblastic tumors(malignant) (n=48)	
Choriocarcinoma	45
Placental site trophoblastic tumor(PSTT)	3
Epithelioid trophoblastic tumor(ETT)	0
Trophoblastic tumor-like lesions (benign)	0
("syncytial endometritis")	6
Placental site nodule	0

Placental site trophoblastic tumor (PSTT)

In 1976, Kurman et al. described 12 patients with a variant of trophoblastic disease marked by a distinct and exaggerated placental site reaction 101. The term "trophoblastic pseudotumor of the uterus" was coined to reflect the apparently benign nature of the lesion. Twiggs et al. 102 reported the death of a young woman with metastatic trophoblastic pseudotumor. In 1981 Scully and Young published a reappraisal of these rare tumors and suggested the term "placental site trophoblastic tumor" (PSTT) to emphasize the potentially malignant nature of the lesion 103.

Clinical findings

PSTT may complicate or follow normal pregnancy, abortion or hydatidiform mole. The symptoms can appear from weeks up to 15 years after termination of pregnancy. Most patients present with irregular vaginal bleeding 104. PSTT presents with metastases in about 10% of cases and metastases are found to develop in an additional 10% during follow up. Although the majority of patients with non-metastatic PSTT are cured by hysterectomy, a number of cases require aggressive treatment with chemotherapy and/or radiation 105.

Gross

In most cases, the tumor is circumscribed and may project as polypoid mass in the uterine cavity or mainly involve the myometrium. The tumor is soft, tan brown and often shows foci of hemorrhages and necrosis. It can extend up to the uterine serosa and may involve adenexa, broad ligament or other organ like large bowel (Figure 28 A, B).

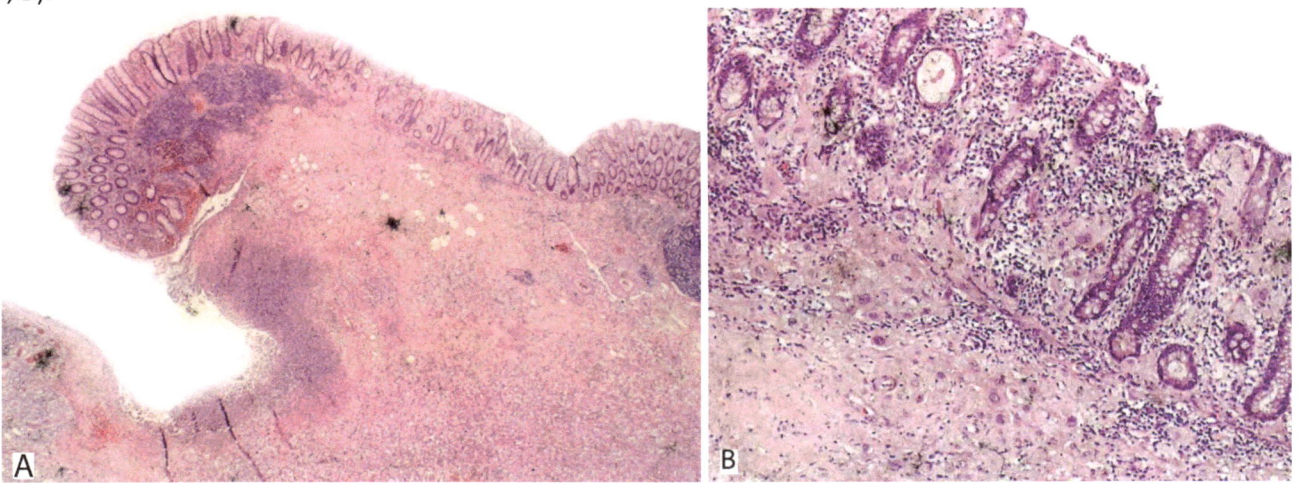

Microscopic

PSTT is composed of large polyhedral implantation site intermediate trophoblastic cells with irregular hyperchromatic nuclei and dense eosinophilic cytoplasm. Most of the cell population is monomorphic in contrast to mixture of cytotrophoblast, intermediate trophoblastic cell and syncitial trophoblastic cell seen in choriocarcinoma. The cells are arranged in cohesive sheets, groups and cords and freely infiltrate between muscle fibers (Figure 28 C) and characteristically replace vessels walls. In about 10% of cases, the tumor is quite aggressive and shows prominent nuclear anaplasia, particularly in case with metastatic disease (Figure 28 D). The case illustrated here represents a case of placental site trophoblastic tumor in uterus with extension to rectum.

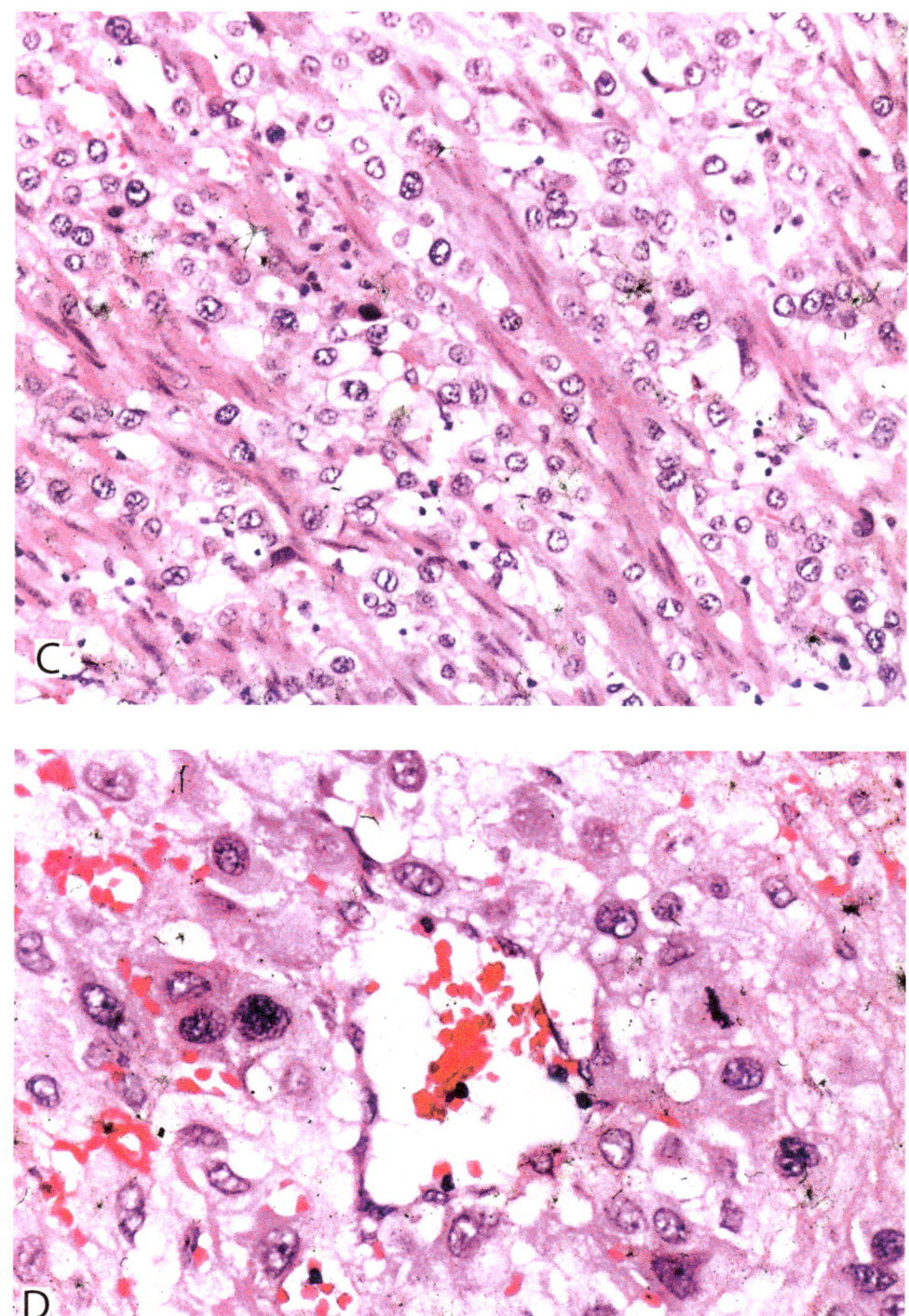

Figure 28 Placental site trophoblastic tumor involving rectal wall (A) scanner view; (B) low power view; (C) Isolated tumor cells permeating between smooth muscle cells; (D) florid nuclear anaplasia in a case, which metastasized to liver

Differential Diagnosis

PSTT can be differentiated from gestational choriocarcinoma by its monomorphic cell population, lack of necrosis and hemorrhage. The beta HCG values are often low and certainly well below the levels encountered in choriocarcinoma. Immunohistochemical studies demonstrate variable reactivity, with only few cells staining for human chorionic gonadotropin and the majority expressing human placental lactogen. 104, 106

Exaggerated placental site reaction(synonymous with "Syncitial endometritis")

This is defined as excess proliferation of implantation site intermediate trophoblasts, which infiltrate the endometrium and myometrium. Some of these cells are multinucleated.

The diagnosis of an exaggerated placental site is rather difficult , since both, this lesion and PSTT are characterized by proliferation of intermediate trophoblasts with infiltration in the myometrium. Both the lesions also show identical immunophenotype. Confluent sheets of trophoblastic cells, typical mitotic Figures, and absence of chorionic villi are diagnostic of PSTT. The exaggerated placental site is a small sized lesion (<5 mm), shows no mitotic activity and presents mixture of decidua and chorionic villi. One more useful criterion is significantly elevated Ki-67 labeling index (>10%) in PSTT but near zero in normal and exaggerated placental site 107.

Placental Site Nodule/Plaque (PSN-P)

This is another major lesion that should be distinguished from PSTT. It is characterized by its relatively small size, circumscription, extensive hyalinization, degenerative features and lack of mitosis 108.

Prognosis of PSTT

Although the majority of patients with non- metastatic PSTT are cured by hysterectomy, a number of cases require aggressive treatment with chemotherapy and/or radiation 105. According to Goldstein 104 early diagnosis and effective treatment of patients with gestational trophoblastic neoplasia has resulted in 100 percent cure rates in non-metastatic disease and in the majority of patients with metastases. In an analysis of 88 cases, the outcomes of patients with FIGO stage I–II disease after hysterectomy were excellent; while those with FIGO stage III–IV diseases had an only 30% survival 109

Tumors of the Ovary

Table 6: Ovarian Tumors (n=2244) Author's series (1970-2006)		
Serous tumors (n=778)		
	Cystadenoma	467 (60%)
	Borderline	34 (4.4%)
	Carcinoma	277 (35.6%)
Mucinous tumors (n=342)		
	Cystadenoma	266 (77.7%)
	Borderline	17 ((5%)
	Carcinoma	59 (17.2%)
Endometrioid tumors (n=136)		
	Cystadenoma	03 (2.2%)
	Borderline	00
	Carcinoma	133 (98.8%)
Clear cell tumor (n=11)		
	Carcinoma	11
Transitional cell tumors (n=8)		
	Brenner tumor (One with mucinous cystadenoma)	6
	Brenner, malignant	2
	Transitional cell carcinoma	1
	Squamous cell carcinoma	5
Sex Cord Stromal tumors (n=185)		
	Granulosa cell	63
	Juvenile granulosa	2
	Thecoma	72
	Fibroma	24
	Sclerosing stromal	6
	Sertoli-Leydig cell	9
	Sex cord annular tubules	2
	Sex cord stromal (NOS)	2
	Hilus cell tumor	4
	Steroid cell	1
Germ Cell Tumors (n=652)		
	Dysgerminoma	52
	Gonadoblastoma	3
	Embryonal carcinoma	4
	Endodermal sinus tumor	30
	Benign cystic teratoma	512
	Teratoma, mature solid	19
	Struma ovarii	14
	Teratoma with carcinoid	3
	Mixed germ cell tumors	15
Miscellaneous Tumors (n=132)		
	Leiomyoma (fibroid)	45
	Leiomyosarcoma	2
	MMMT	13
	Adenosarcoma (Mullerian)	4
	Mal. Mesenchymoma	2
	Metastatic carcinoma	66

Surface Epithelial Tumors

Surface epithelium also called germinal epithelium or coelomic epithelium undergoes Mullerian differentiation, as a result of which it can produce any of the adult structures formed by the Mullerian ducts. The epithelial tumors are classified according to their putative histogenesis: serous, (tubal) mucinous (endocervical), endometrioid, clear cell, Brenner/transitional cell etc. Mixtures of different cell types occur commonly and some are undifferentiated and hence unclassifiable. Epithelial tumors comprise about 60% of all ovarian neoplasms and more than 90% of the malignant tumors. As per WHO classification, all epithelial tumors are categorized into benign, borderline and malignant. The histological identification of borderline epithelial tumors may be difficult and study of many sections is required for proper assessment 110-112. In this section, borderline serous and mucinous tumors are discussed at length and illustrated adequately.

Serous borderline tumors (SBT) Synonyms:

Synonyms Serous ovarian tumors of low malignant potential, atypical proliferating serous tumor, cystadenoma of borderline malignancy

Definition:

Ovarian tumor exhibits an epithelial proliferation of serous type of cells, greater than that seen in the benign counterparts but without destructive stromal invasion. About 9 to 15% of all serous neoplasms fall within the borderline category.

Clinical Findings

SBT is most common in 4th and 5th decade, and 30-50% are bilateral. Approximately, 60% are in stage I. In our experience, patients are more commonly detected in the third decade, where fertility preservation is an important consideration.

Gross:

Most SBTs are cystic and solid. The solid areas are whitish and firm, rather than solid and friable as in serous carcinoma, and may have adenofibromatous structure. A borderline serous tumor should be suspected, when tan colored papillary excrescences are seen either within the cyst and / or on the ovarian surface. The contents of the cystic portion are usually serous. In most cases of SBT, the specimen always shows a large predominantly multicystic tumor (Figure 29). If solid friable areas are seen, the index of suspicion for malignancy is high.

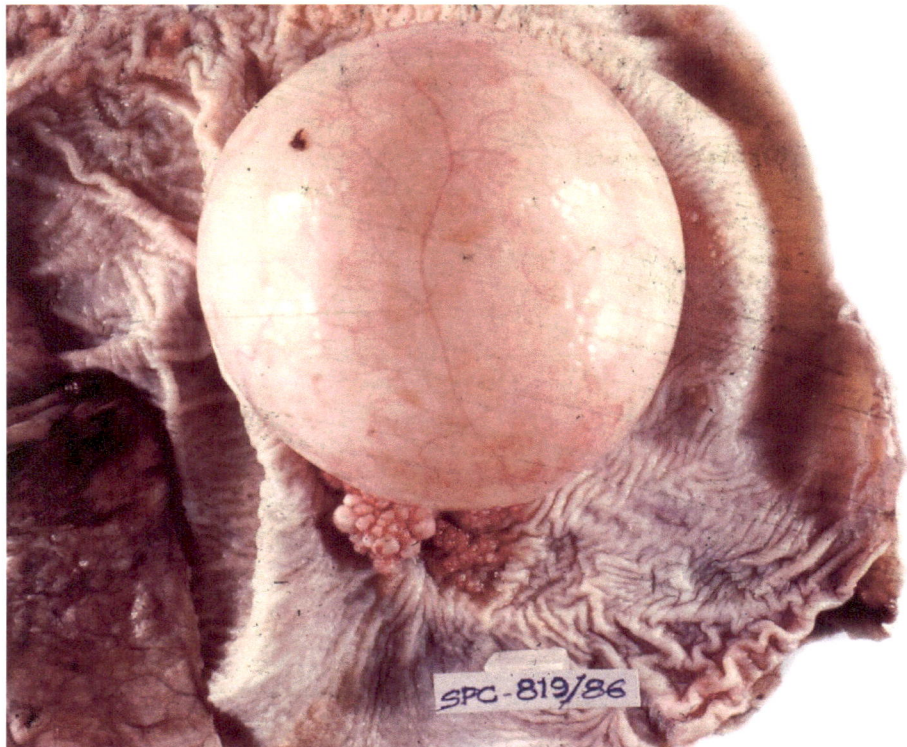

Figure 29 Gross photograph of borderline serous tumor which is predominantly cystic Note focal tiny papillary nodules

Microscopic

The tumor shows papillary proliferation of polygonal or hobnail serous type cells, supported by delicate fibro vascular core. The nuclear atypia is mild or at the most moderate, and mitoses are rare. The papillae show hierarchical branching towards progressively smaller papillae. By definition, there is no stromal invasion.

Some serous cystadenomas have focal epithelial proliferation and atypia. It has been suggested that 10% of the epithelial component should show proliferation and tufting, to call the tumor SBT. Another useful criteria is to look for detached or floating clusters of cells in the lumina to distinguish between cystadenoma and a SBT (Figure 30 A-F) 110, 111, 112

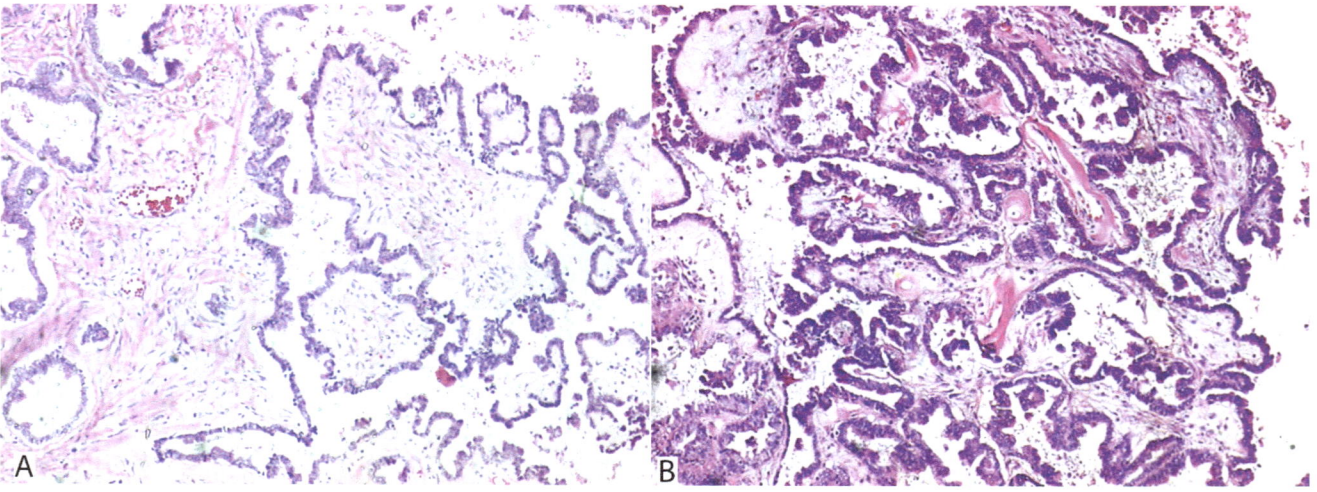

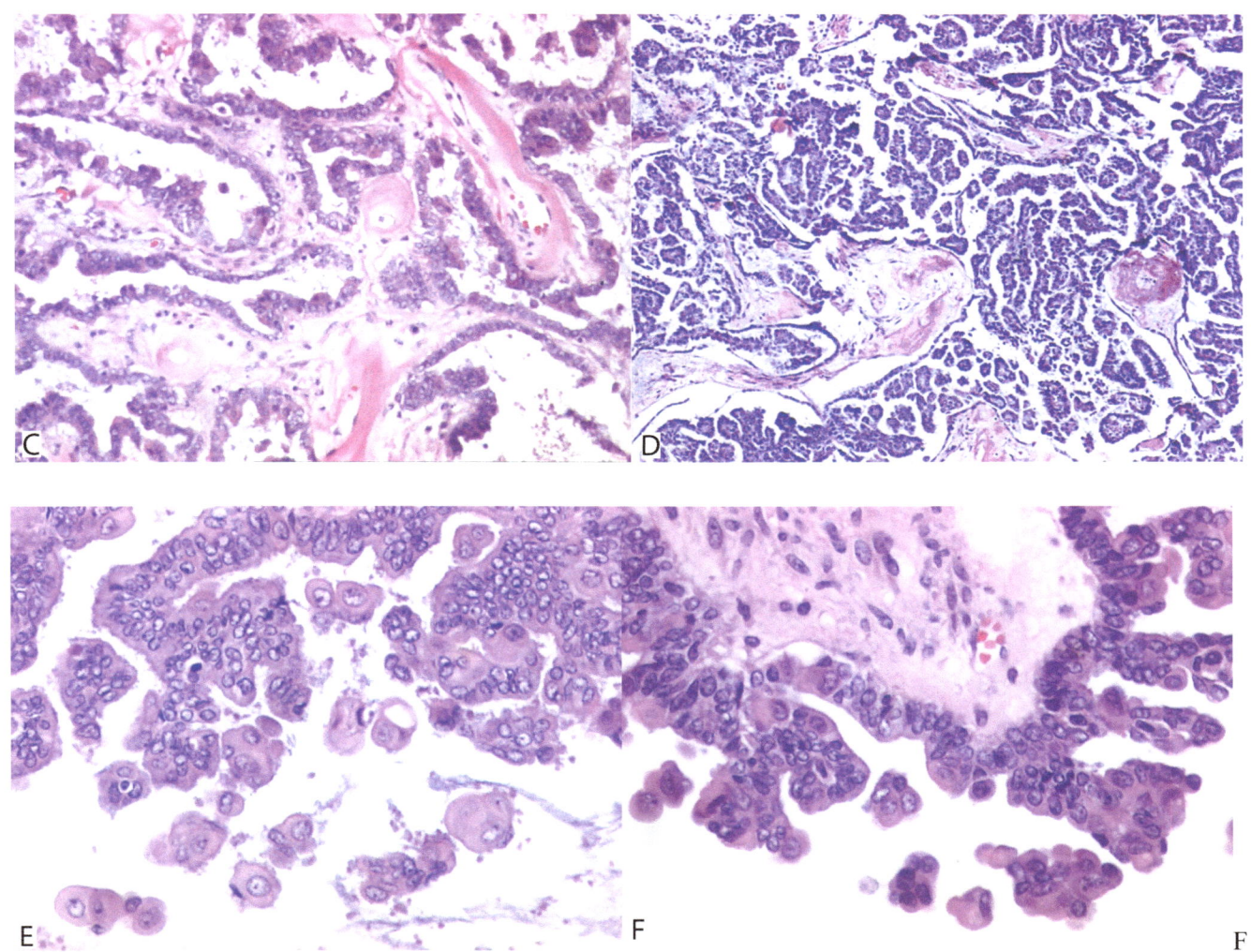

Figure 30. (A-F) Serous borderline tumor of the ovary: epithelial proliferation with papillary architecture (A, B) low power view; (C, D) medium power view showing complex epithelial proliferation; (E, F) detached cell clusters in the cyst lumen with cytological atypia

Serous borderline tumors with microinvasion

About 10-15% of borderline serous tumors show evidence of microinvasion. However these tumors still exhibit favorable prognosis irrespective of the subtype. Histologically, microinvasion is characterized by either single cells with abundant eosinophilic cytoplasm or nests of neoplastic cells that occasionally form a micropapillary or cribriform pattern surrounded by clear clefts. These foci should occupy an area of less than 2-5 mm in each of the two dimensions. Microinvasion is an uncommon finding; and often it is our experience that, even after a generous sampling, a repetitive proliferation pattern without stromal invasion is seen in SBT (Figure 31 A-C) [113,114].

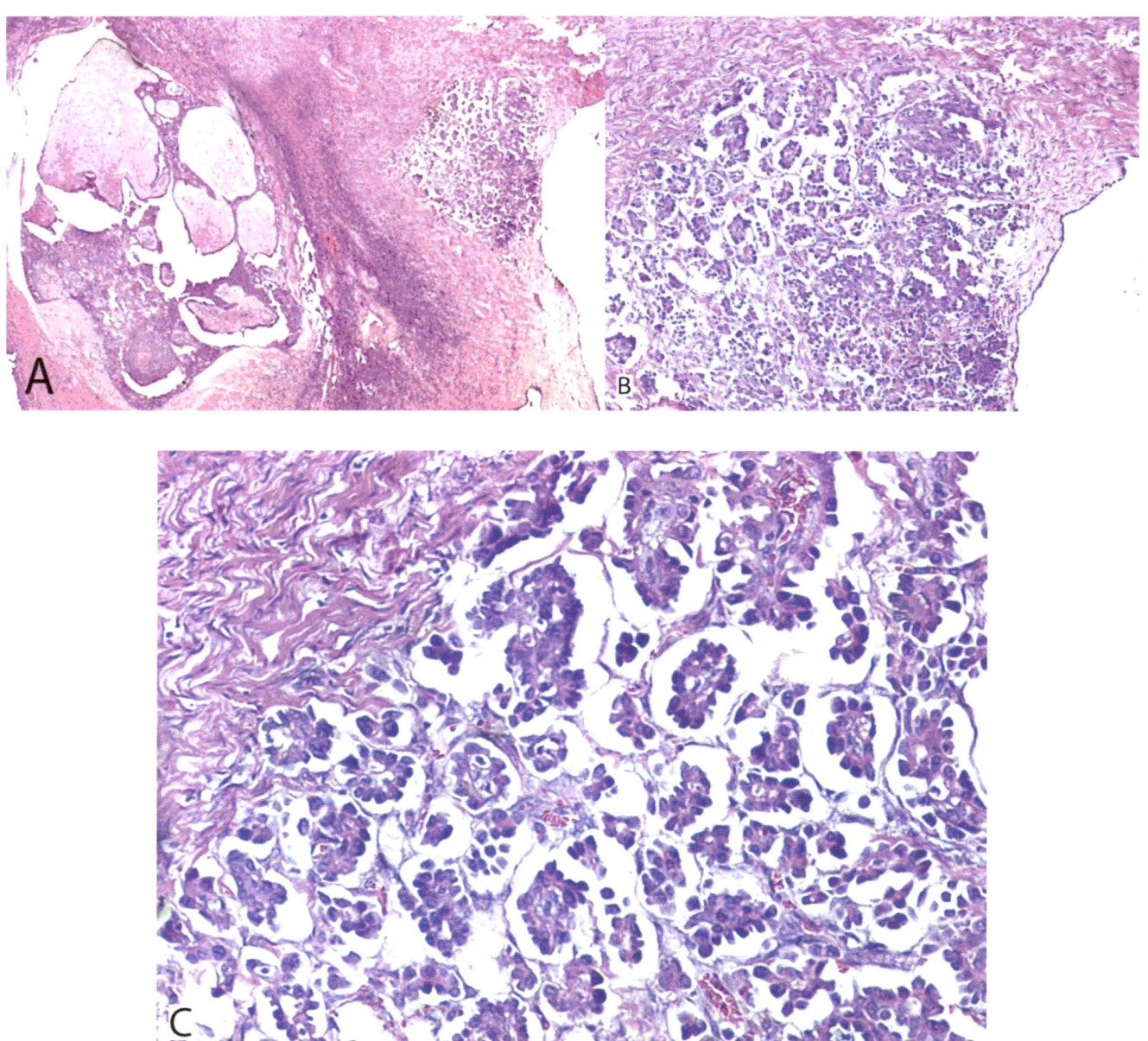

Figure 31 (A) Scanner view of SBT with microinvasion (arrows); (B) microinvasion at low power; (C) microinvasion at high power

About 30-40% of borderline serous tumors are known to be associated with peritoneal and omental implants, which occur at the sites of endosalpingosis. These are divided into non-invasive and invasive implants. The non-invasive implants may be of desmoplastic type or epithelial type. While, the non-invasive implants have no bearing on long term survival, the invasive implants are prognostically important, in that, they are associated with poorer prognosis.

More than 50% cases with invasive implants have recurrences and the 10 - survival rate is only about 35%. The distinction between invasive and non- invasive implants is based on invasion of the adjoining normal tissue such as omental fat or any organ in the vicinity. Invasive implants also would show more cytological atypia. At the time of diagnosis, about 20-40% of SBT are associated with peritoneal implants (PIs)

'SBT with micropapillary pattern' or is it micropapillary carcinoma?

Exuberant and delicate micropapillary proliferation without destructive stromal invasion has been described and designated as micropapillary serous carcinoma by some. Similar lesions with stromal invasion have been termed as micropapillary low grade serous carcinomas. On morphology, they show marked cellular proliferation and mild, uniform cellular atypia. The papillae are typically slender and the term micropapillary is used when the papillae are 5 times longer than their breadth. A non hierarchial branching of papillae is seen, i.e. arising directly from a cyst wall (Figure 32 A-C). However, the designation of micropapillary carcinoma without identifying stromal invasion has not been accepted by many (including WHO 115, 116) . Seidman and Kurman 117 studied 65 advanced stage cases of apparent SBTs and subclasified them as follows:

1) SBT with noninvasive implants (51 cases): follow up 5 & 10 year survival of 98%
2) SBT with invasive implants (3 cases): 10 year survival of 33%
3) SBT with micropapillary pattern (11 cases): 5 year survival of 81% and 10 year survival 71%

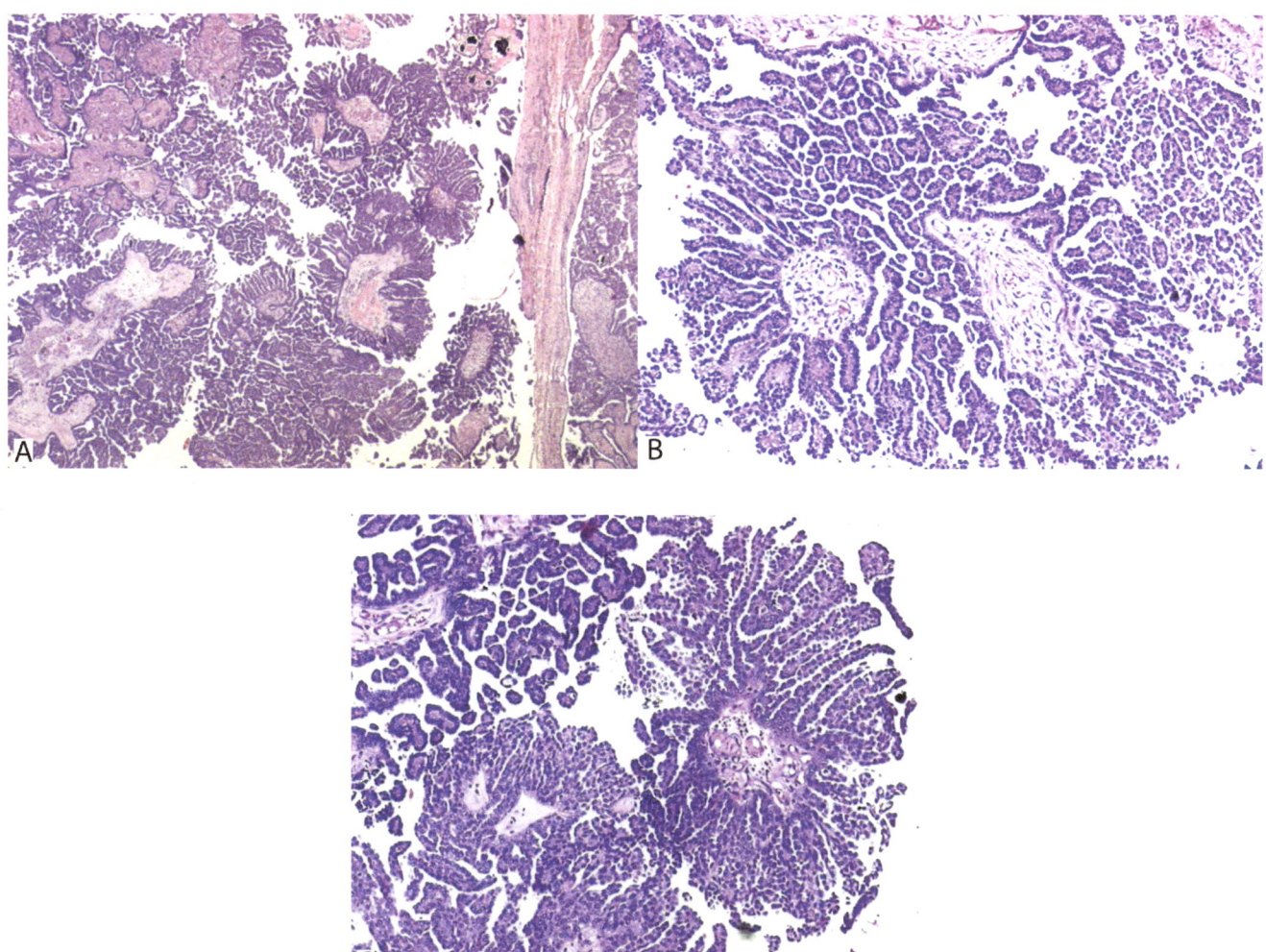

Figure 32 SBT with micro papillary pattern: (A) scanner view; (B, C) medium power views

On the basis of follow up data of 11 cases of SBT micropapillary pattern the authors concluded that this lesion should be designated as micropapillary carcinoma even without the presence of invasive implants. As such, this lesion has better prognosis than conventional invasive serous papillary carcinoma. There is no unanimity about the final call on this matter, whether the process is a low grade carcinoma or SBT with good prognosis. Larger series of cases with careful histological analysis and at least a good 10 year follow up may produce an acceptable conclusion. The authors' practice is to designate such tumors as serous borderline tumors with micropapillary pattern (and qualify implants, if seen, as they are), rather than the label of micropapillary serous carcinoma.

Serous borderline tumors with lymph node involvement

It is difficult to comprehend as to how an ovarian serous tumor with lymph node metastasis can be still designated as a borderline tumor rather than a carcinoma. This requires an understanding of a benign condition called endosalpingosis, which is most commonly observed in the peritoneum, omentum and ovary in 5% to 25% of females. It is characterized by small cysts or simple papillae lined by cytologically benign bland ciliated columnar cells of tubal epithelial type. Psammoma bodies may be seen and in some fibrosis with chronic inflammation occurs in the inclusions. These benign inclusions, also called Mullerian epithelial inclusions, have been described in pelvic lymph nodes and pelvic peritoneal surface (Figure 33 A-D).

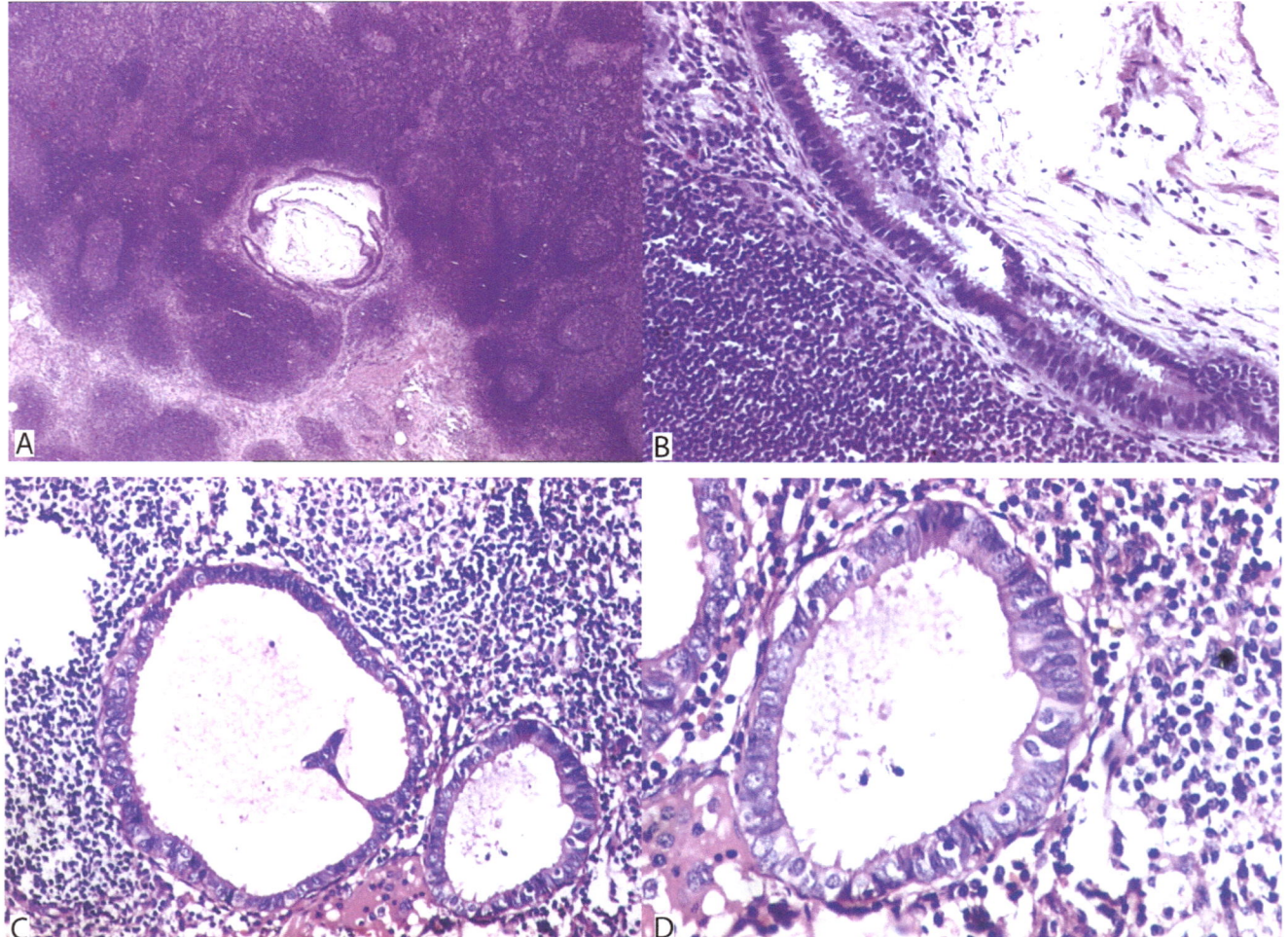

Figure 33 Benign Mullerian inclusions in a lymph node: (A) scanner view; (B) Low power view; (C, D). The glands are isolated and may be found accidentally within the pelvic lymph nodes.

A study of benign glandular inclusions in autopsy and surgical materials from both males and females has been carried out. The inclusions were found in 19 of 128 (14.8%) specimens from females but none from males. It was concluded that the inclusions were benign and exclusively found in females.

SBT can involve pelvic and para-aortic lymph nodes and occasionally extra-abdominal lymph nodes. Foci of endosalpingosis usually occur within the capsule or fibrous trabeculae in lymph nodes. Such inclusions are seen more commonly in patients with SBT, and papillary proliferation are found arising from benign inclusions, like in peritoneal implants. In a series of 43 cases of SBT with lymph node metastasis, the reported survival rate was 98%. Thus, involvement of pelvic and abdominal nodes by SBT does not appear to indicate an adverse prognosis.

There has been a debate about lymph node dissection in cases of SBT; some oncologists do not carry out lymph node dissection and some do. It has been proposed that SBT involving nodes may represent separate foci of synchronous growth rather than true metastasis. In conclusion, the designation SBT has been retained for cases of SBT with lymph node metastasis because the survival rate is so high and survival rate for conventional serous carcinoma a poor 45% 118,119,120.

Prognosis

The behavior of SBT with microinvasion is similar to that of SBT. Unilateral salpingo-oophorectomy is acceptable therapy for younger women who wish to preserve fertility.

Surgical pathological stage and type of extra ovarian disease are the most important prognostic factors in SBT. The overall disease free survival for Stage I SBT is 99.5%. Survival for advanced stage disease with noninvasive implants is 95.3% and that for survival of tumors with invasive implants is 66% 117, 121, 122.

Serous Carcinomas of Ovary

Concept of Type I (low grade carcinoma) and type II (high grade carcinoma)

It is now accepted that there are two distinct types of ovarian serous carcinomas- low grade and high grade, on the basis of biological behavior. It is to be clarified that they are not two grades of the same neoplasm; but represent two different entities with differing pathogenesis, molecular events, behavior and prognosis.

Type I serous low grade carcinomas, serous cystadenoma, SBT, SBT with micropapillary areas form a continuous spectrum. Low grade carcinoma is thought to arise from cystadenoma, through borderline serous tumor - borderline serous tumor with micropapillary pattern and then invasive low grade carcinoma (similar to a well- defined adenoma carcinoma sequence in colo-rectum). Low grade carcinomas show <12 mitoses per 10 HPF and do not show necrosis or multinucleated tumor giant cells. Type II high grade carcinomas are more common than the low grade carcinomas. Necrosis, multinucleated giant cells and mitoses >12 per 10 HPF are typically seen in this cancer.

High grade carcinomas are aggressive, show initial response to chemotherapy therapy but exhibit recurrence and are eventually fatal 123,124.

Type I Carcinoma	Type II Carcinoma
KRAS or *BRAF* mutations-no p53 mutations	No *KRAS* or *BRAF* mutations
lower expression of MIB-1, bcl2,	Higher expression of p53, bcl2, MIB-1, p16
Low expression of Her-2neu, p16.	Higher expression of Her-2neu
Weak or negative expression for p53	p53 mutation, high chromosomal instability
Both express WT1	Both express WT1
Express ER (Possible therapeutic role)	May express ER (weakly)

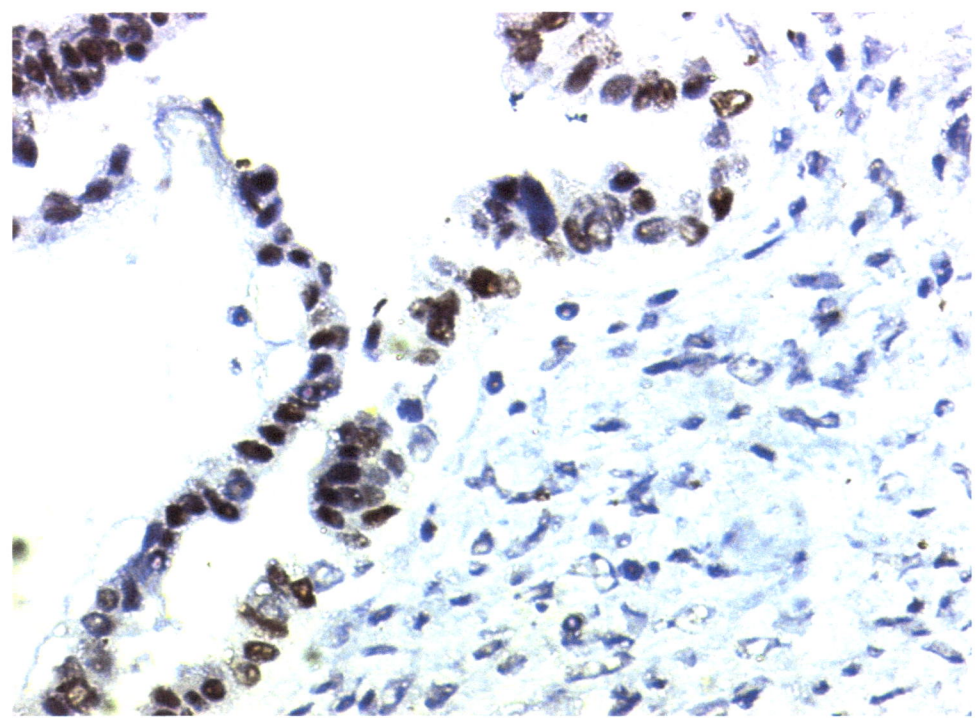

Figure 34 Serous Carcinoma of Ovary: ER positivity in Low grade serous carcinoma

Mucinous borderline tumors

Mucinous tumors of the ovary are defined as those where some or all of the epithelial cells contain intracytoplasmic mucin. The cells may resemble those of endocervix, gastric pylorus or intestine. In some tumors only scattered goblet cells are present, in an epithelium that is otherwise non mucinous.

Mucinous cystadenoma, cystadenofibroma, borderline mucinous tumor and cystadenocarcinoma are the mucinous tumor types that are recognized. Mucinous tumors account for 12%-15% of all ovarian tumors. The vast majority of them are benign (75%), 10% borderline, 15% carcinomas 125,126.

Mucinous Borderline Tumors

(MBT Synonyms- Mucinous tumors of low malignant potential, mucinous tumors of borderline malignancy

Definition

These ovarian tumors are of low malignant potential, exhibiting proliferation of mucinous type cells greater than that seen in their benign counterparts but without stromal invasion (Figure 35 A, B).

Two main subtypes (intestinal type constituting 85%-90% of mucinous borderline tumors, and endocervical or Mullerian type, accounting for remaining 10%-15% of MBTs) are identified.

MBT of intestinal type

The tumors are usually large and multiloculated, containing watery to viscous mucoid material. They are usually unilateral, and have no tendency to form extra-ovarian implants or lymph node metastases.

Microscopic

Areas resembling mucinous cystadenomas (single layered mucinous epithelium with no atypia) are common. However, in the borderline areas, cell stratification and papillary architecture is seen; occasional mitotic Figures are present (Figure 35 A, B). The cytological atypia is mild or at most moderate in nature. Goblet cells and sometimes Paneth cells or even neuroendocrine cells with intracytoplasmic eosinophilic granules are seen. At times, rupture of a mucinous gland can result in histiocytic or granulomatous response in the cyst wall (mucin granuloma). This has no adverse effect on prognosis 127,128,129. Extensive mucin deposits in the ovarian stroma, outside the confines of the glands, are called psuedomyxoma ovarii.

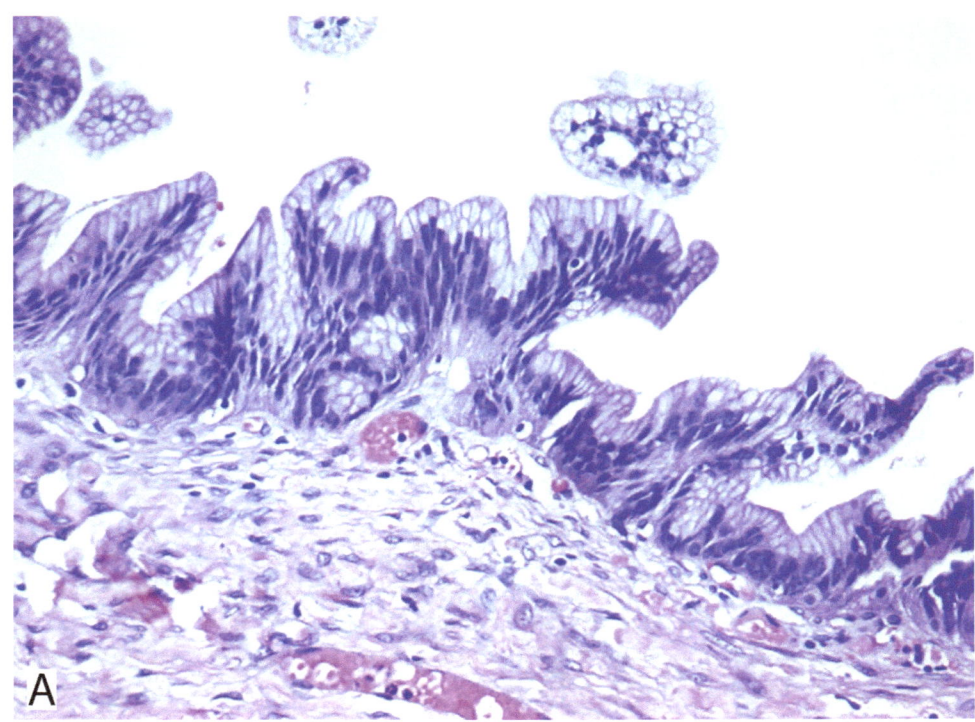

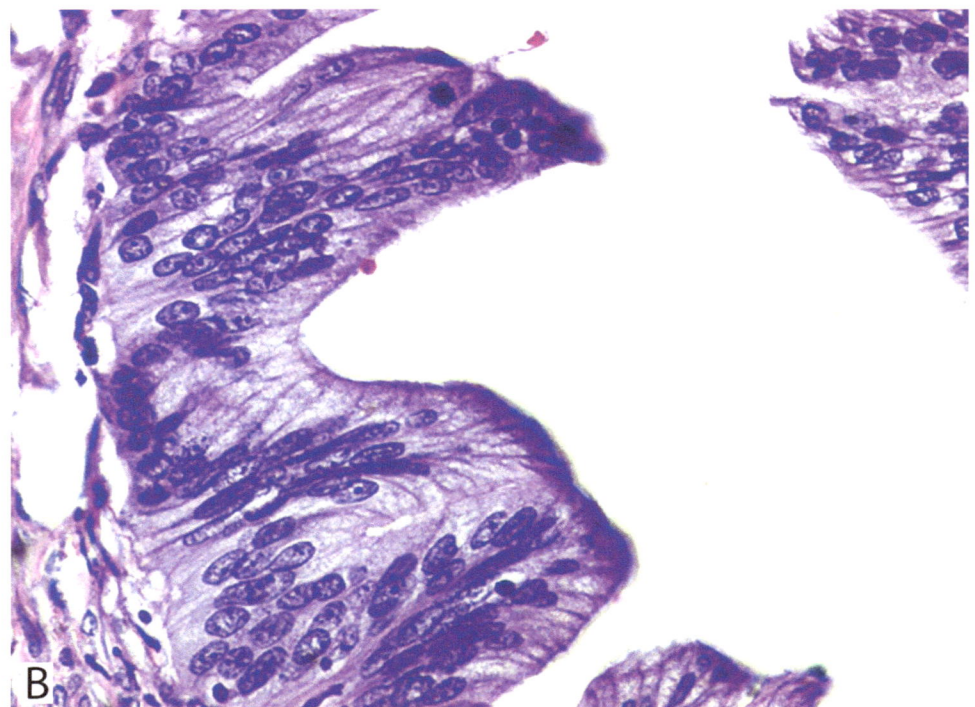

Figure 35 Borderline mucinous tumor: (A) nuclear stratification and mild nuclear atypia; (B) medium power view showing an occasional mitotic Figure)

Intraepithelial carcinoma and microinvasion in intestinal MBT

Intraepithelial carcinoma or intramucosal carcinoma is the term used when the cytological atypia is of severe degree. Complex/ florid epithelial proliferation, but without severe cytological atypia, does not qualify for a diagnosis of intraepithelial carcinoma (where MBT designation is appropriate).

As with serous tumors, a category of microinvasion is recognized, most using 3 mm size criteria. Its clinical significance is not firmly established.

Endocervical type (Mullerian type) MBT are often associated with endometriosis, much less common than intestinal type, bilateral in 20%-40% of cases, and smaller in size than intestinal type. Low power may show papillary appearance, but the lining cells contain cytoplasmic mucin (resembling endocervical type epithelium).At times, squamous elements or foci resembling serous epithelial lining are seen, when a designation of seromucinous tumor is used. Neutrophils are often seen in the stroma which is a useful diagnostic feature. It has been found that foci of microinvasion and intraepithelial carcinoma do not have adverse effect on prognosis 130.

MBT: ovarian primary or metastatic mucinous carcinoma

It is increasingly recognized that majority of the borderline mucinous ovarian tumors, do in fact, represent metastasis from inapparent or dormant primary sites like appendix and rarely in other gastrointestinal tract sites; and at the time of making this diagnosis, such a primary may not be known to be present.

Primary mucinous borderline tumors of the ovary do exist; but some pathologists append a comment in the report that primary elsewhere may be excluded on clinical or imaging grounds before accepting that this as a primary MBT. In a review of 22 cases of mucinous tumors involving appendix and ovary, 21 cases were synchronous and typically similar histologically, with features similar to those of cystadenomas and MBTs. This study has shown that diagnosis of metastatic mucinous tumor in ovary is based on a constellation of findings: typical synchronous presentation of ovarian and appendiceal tumors, their histological similarity, frequency of bilateral ovarian mucinous tumors and the usual presence of mucin and atypical mucinous cells on the ovarian surface 131,132. If, an ovarian tumor is suspected to be a mucinous tumor, either on imaging grounds or as an intraoperative finding, then appendicectomy is recommended. The surgical pathologist should submit the entire appendix {multiple transverse sections) for a complete histological study, even if no gross lesion is identified.

Pseudomyxoma Peritonei (PMP)

PMP is a poorly understood condition characterized by mucinous ascites and mucinous implants diffusely involving the peritoneal surfaces. Pseudomyxoma Peritonei in women may be ovarian or appendiceal in origin, with cases of appendiceal origin accounting for the majority of cases. Appendiceal origin can be excluded with certainty after microscopic examination of the appendix has disclosed it to be normal. When the appendix and ovary are involved, the appendiceal tumor is probably primary and the ovarian tumor secondary. The link between mucinous tumors of the appendix, borderline ovarian mucinous tumors and PMP in the same patient is mysterious but has been reported by many. The ovary and appendix are not closely related embryologically or functionally. It is possible that they are subject to similar oncogenic process, but is not obvious why this should be so 133.

PMP encompass two distinct entities:

(i) 125 disseminated peritoneal adenomucinosis, which is an indolent proliferation of morphologically benign or minimally atypical "adenomatous" epithelium nearly always derived from a ruptured mucinous appendiceal adenomatous tumor. Histologically it is characterized by pools of mucin with scanty or focally proliferative mucinous epithelium having mild atypia. The patients with disseminated peritoneal adenomucinosis have prolonged survival, but eventually succumb to complications of bowel obstruction. According to one view these tumors are not true carcinomas, but represent a very low grade, clinically indolent neoplasm that needs to be distinguished from the aggressive peritoneal mucinous carcinomatosis (Figure 36 A-F).

(ii) 126 peritoneal mucinous carcinomatosis, which is a high grade metastatic adenocarcinoma usually arising from appendix or colon with a high early mortality. In these cases, the peritoneal lesions are composed of more abundant mucinous epithelium with architectural and cytoplasmic features of carcinoma (Figure 37 A-F).

DIAGNOSTIC PROBLEMS IN TUMORS OF FEMALE GENITAL TRACT: SELECTED TOPICS

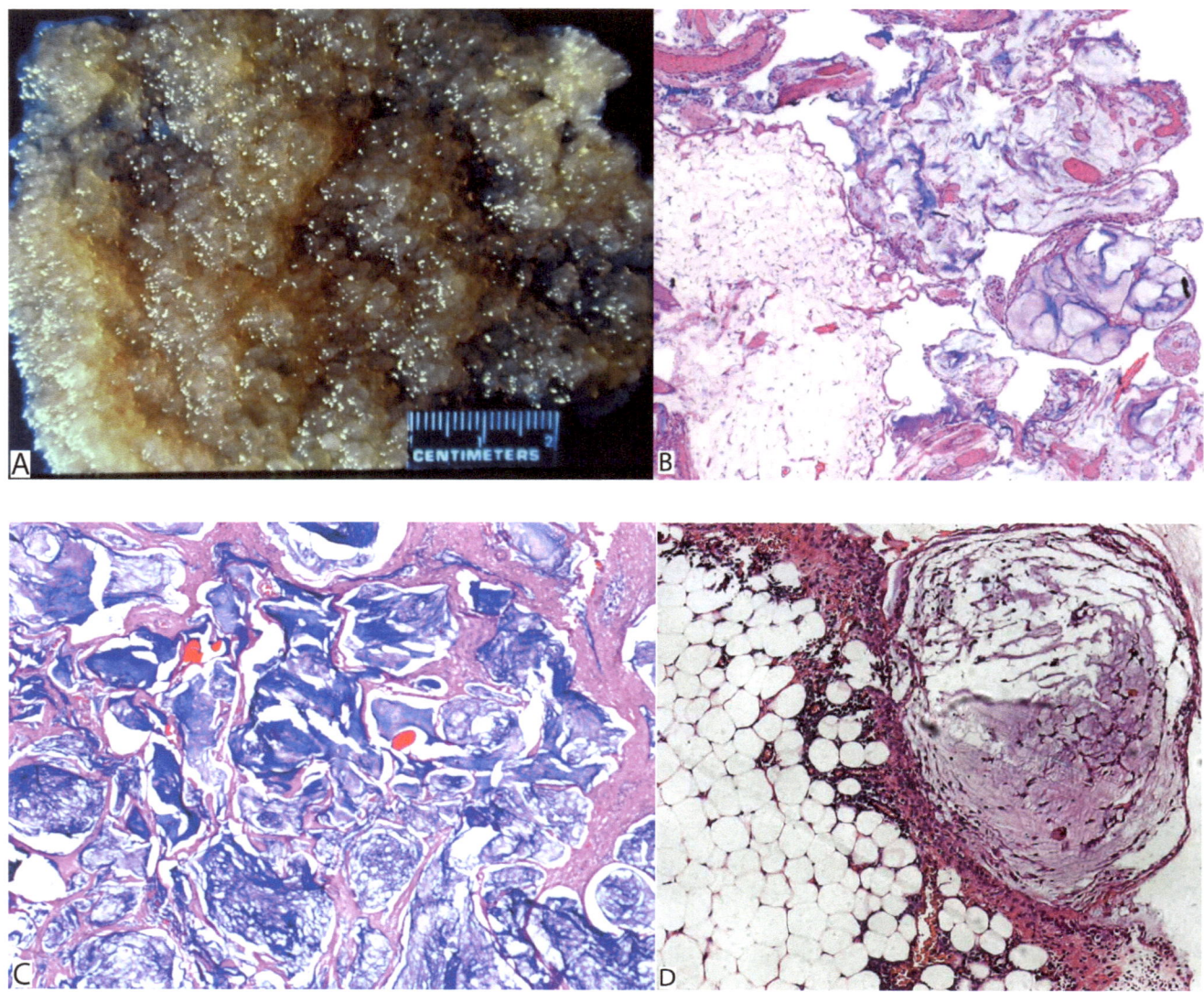

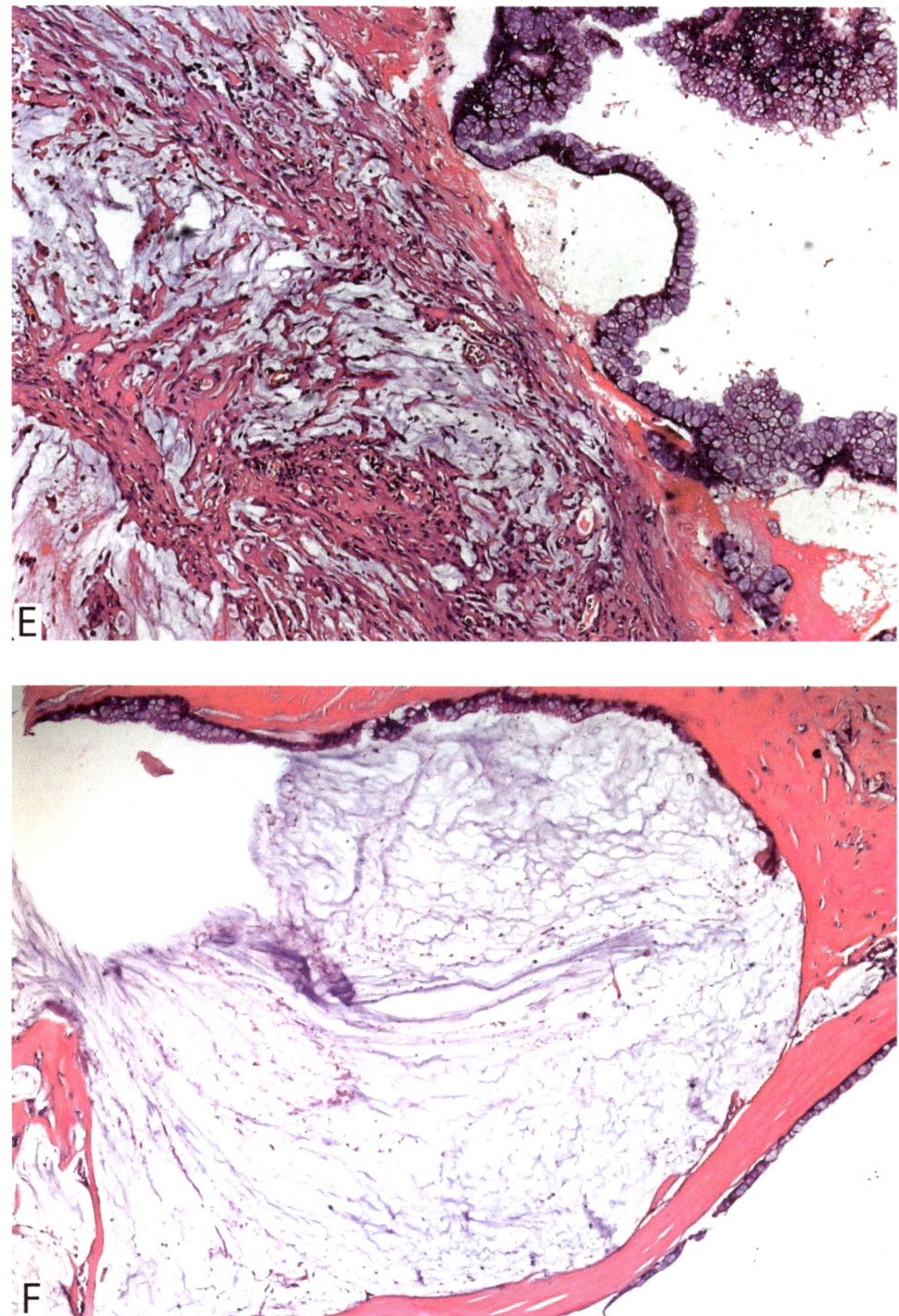

Figure 36 A case of disseminated peritoneal adenomucinosis (A) Gross appearance of pseudomyxomaperitonei: note sheets of mucinous globules with no solid tumorous lesion; (B,C, D) lobulated masses of mucoid material on the surface of omental peritoneum with no mucinous epithelium; (E, F) strips of benignmucinous epithelium in monolayer with no nuclear anaplasia, note many thick bands of fibrosis in the mucinous backdrop in E

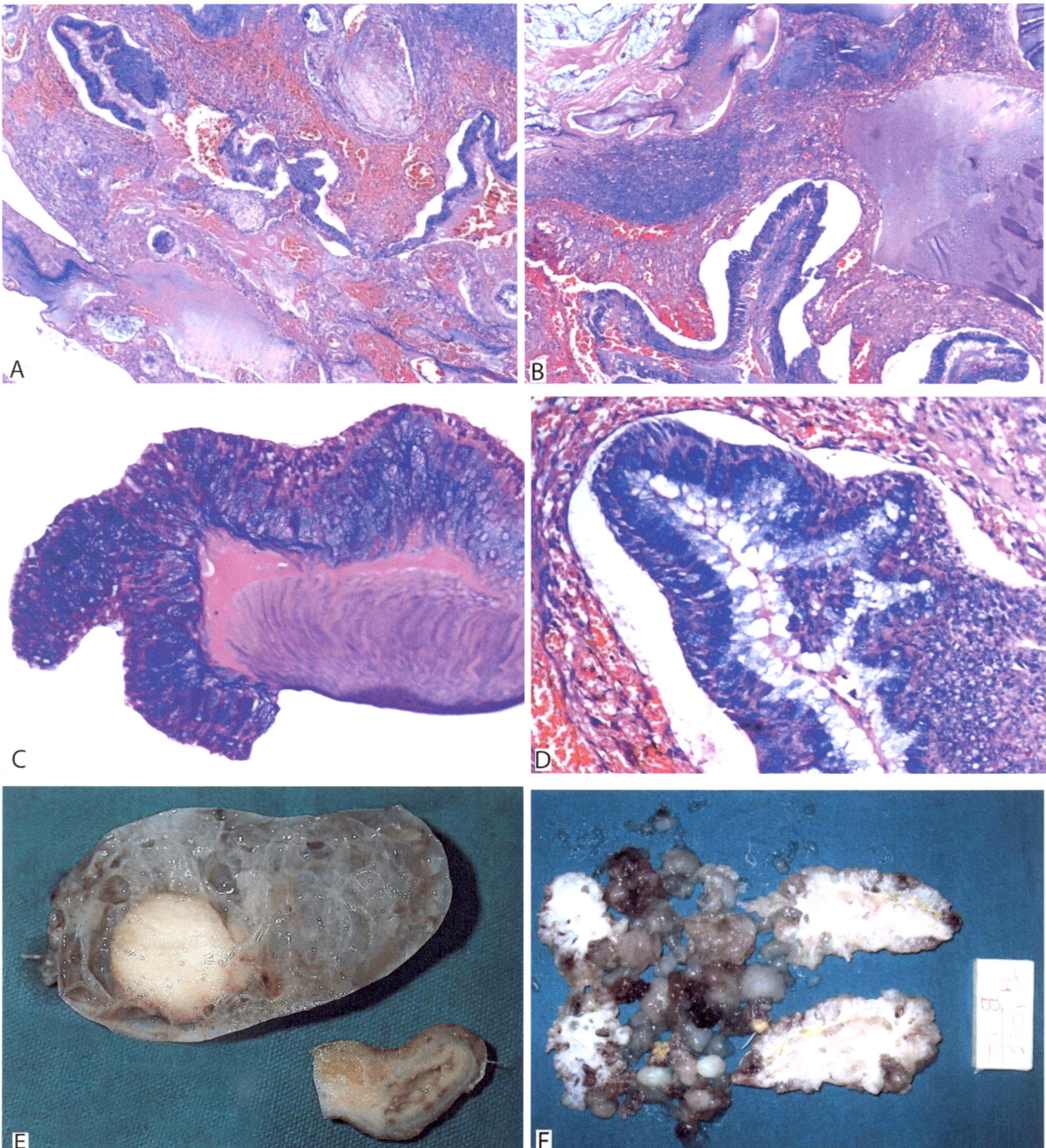

Figure 37 A case of well differentiated adenocarcinoma of appendix with peritoneal mucinous carcinomatosis (A,B) low power view of metastatic adenocarcinoma on the peritoneal surface. Many thick neoplastic glands and papillae with intimately mixed mucin (C, D) neoplastic gland and a papilla exhibiting stratified enlarged hyperchromatic nuclei; (E) Gross photo of the mucinous appendicular adenocarcinoma with metastatic mucinous ovarian tumor;(F) peritoneal mucinous carcinomatosis

OVARIAN SURFACE EPITHELIAL TUMORS

Immunohistochemistry

IHC has provided supportive evidence that mucinous tumors of ovaries with pseudomyxoma peritonei are derived from associated appendiceal mucinous tumor. These tumors display diffusely positive staining for CK 20 and negative staining for CK 7. In contrast, primary ovarian borderline mucinous tumors are all diffusely positive for CK 7 134. In addition, identical K-ras mutations were demonstrated in the ovarian and appendiceal neoplasms in a series of 16 cases 135.

Clinical Behavior (Prognosis)

Long term follow up data was analyzed for a previously reported series of 109 cases of PMP. Patients with disseminated peritoneal adenomucinosis had a 5 and 10 year survival rate of 75% and 68% (mean follow up 8 years) and patients with peritoneal mucinous carcinomatosis had a 5 and 10 year survival rate of 14% and 3%. In fact, for the latter group more than 90% of patients die within 3 years 136, 137

Clear cell carcinoma of the ovary

This group of tumors possesses a predominant epithelial component containing mainly glycogen filled clear cells, hobnail cells, and rarely other type of cells. A variable fibroblastic stromal component is present. Most of the clear cell neoplasms of the ovaries are carcinomas, clear cell adenofibromas, and borderline tumors are very rare indeed.

Clinical Features

The mean age of the patient is 57 years compared to 64 years median for ovarian serous tumor. CCC is known to be associated with thromboembolic disease (about 40%). It differs from the usual ovarian serous carcinomas in many ways: higher incidence amongst Asian women, younger age, and low stage tumors at presentation (Stage I/II 57% to 81%). The relatively early presentation of this tumor may be related to the associated symptoms of pelvic endometriosis. At operation, endometriotic implants are often seen in close proximity to tumor or elsewhere in the pelvis or abdomen. Amongst all surface epithelial tumors, CCC has the highest association with pelvic endometriosis.

Gross

The tumor is usually spongy, but more commonly shows thick walled unilocular cystic appearance, with multiple fleshy nodules within it. The cysts contain clear watery or mucinous fluid.

Microscopic

CCCs show a variety of morphological patterns such as tubulo-cystic, papillary, solid or combinations of all. The cells are polyhedral with abundant clear cytoplasm, separated by delicate fibro vascular cores. The tubulo-cystic pattern shows hobnail type cells protruding into the lumen. Occasionally, oxyphil cells are noted. Signet ring cells often contain inspissated mucinous material in the center of a vacuole, referred to as ' targetoid' cells. Mucin may be seen in the lumen of the cysts or tubules (Figure 38 A-D).

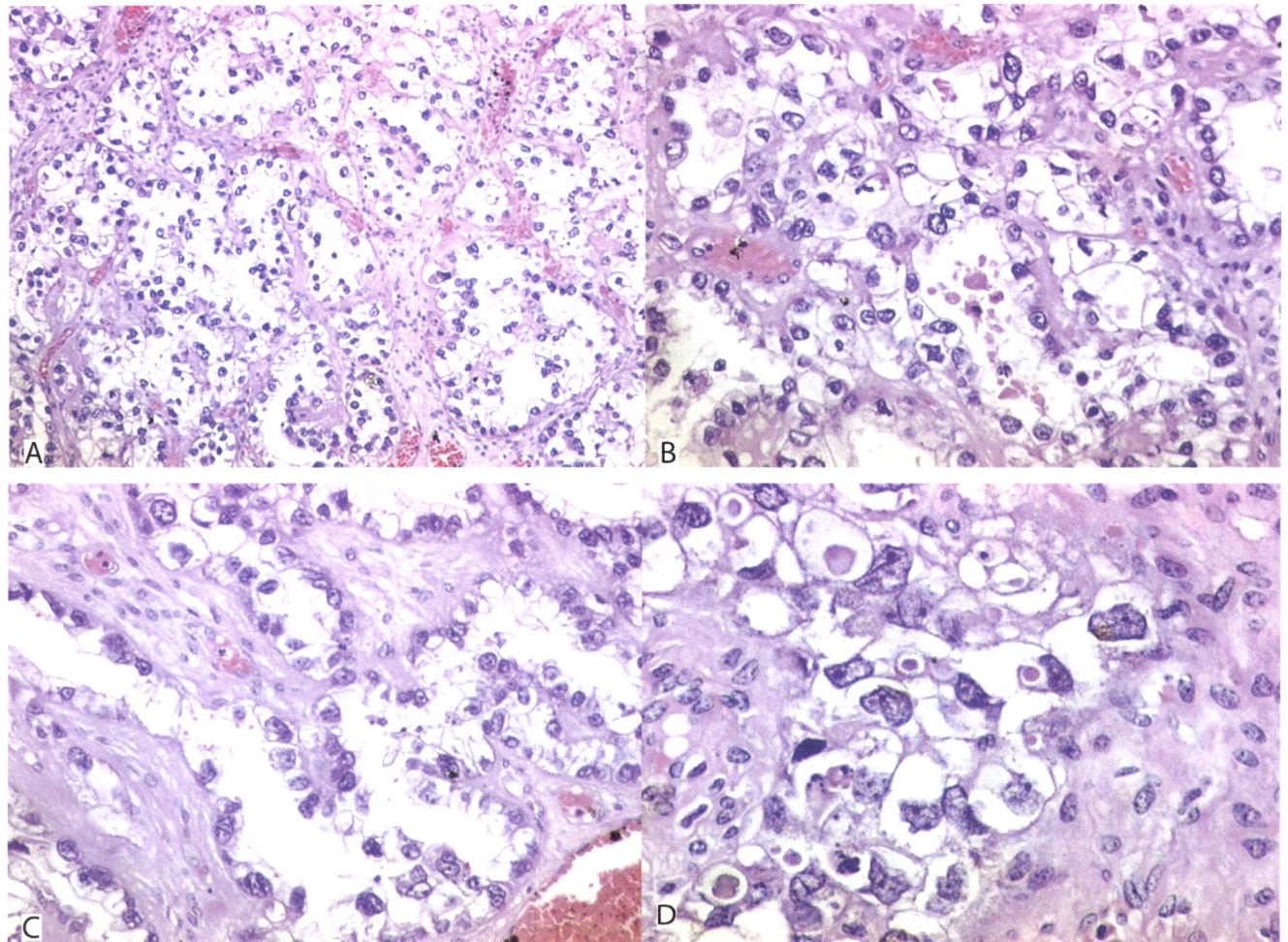

Figure 38 Clear cell carcinoma of the ovary: (A) Low power showing tubular architecture and hobnailing; (B, C) medium power showing nuclear atypia and hobnailing; (D) eosinophilic inclusions are seen in the cytoplasm

Prognosis

When controlled for the stage, ovarian CCCs show lower survival than ovarian serous carcinomas: 5-yr survival 69% for stage I, 55% for stag II, 14% for stage III, and 4% for stage IV. Low survival rates in ovarian CCC may be due to lack of sensitivity to platinum based chemotherapy. This, in turn, may be related to low nuclear proliferation rate in tumor cells and decrease in accumulation of platinum in tumor cells. Response rate to chemotherapy in patients with CCC ranges from 11%-45%, which is lower than for serous carcinoma 138, 139, 140, 141

Differential diagnosis

Ovarian serous carcinoma is positive for WT1, p53, and for ER, PR, while ovarian CCC is negative for these markers. Instead, ovarian CCC is positive for hepatocyte nuclear factor- 1 beta (HNF 1Beta.

Yolk sac tumor is an important differential diagnosis. Preoperative raised serum alpha fetoprotein levels are helpful. Since, YST shows a variety of patterns, morphology may closely mimic CCC. IHC with CK7, Leu M1 (CD15), CA 125 (positive in 50% cases), CEA (positive in 38% cases) is helpful. YST can routinely show cytokeratin positivity, and there are occasional reports with AFP positivity in CCC. Recently, better antibody HNF1 beta is suggested as a marker for CCC of the ovary and glypican 3 is emerging as a much better marker for YST. Hence, a panel of glypican- 3, CK7, LeuM1, CA 125 and HNF1Beta) can be used.

Gonadoblastoma (Germ cell-sex cord-stromal tumor)

Definition

The term Gonadoblastoma may be defined as a neoplasm containing an intimate mixture of germ cells and elements resembling immature granulosa or Sertoli cells; Leydig cells or lutein type cells may or may not be present 142. It almost always arises from a dysgenetic gonad and in the past it has been called dysgenetic gonadoma.

Clinical findings

Gonadoblstomas occur in patients with pure or mixed forms of gonadal dysgenesis, male pseudo hermaphrodites or some related type of intersex condition. In a series of 74 cases, 85% of the patients were phenotypically females, who were commonly virilized, whereas remainder were phenotypically males, who mostly presented with cryptorchidism, hypospadias and female internal secondary sex organs 142. Most patients with gonadoblastoma are phenotypic females with dysgenetic gonads, are chromatin negative, and have 46 XY karyotype. There are four cases of pregnant women with gonadoblastoma, reported in the literature, which indicate that this tumor can occur in functionally and morphologically normal gonads and that occurrence of gonadoblastoma in abnormal gonads is not an absolute rule. About 200 cases of gonadoblastoma have been reported but occurrence of this tumor in fertile women continues to be extremely low 143.

Gross

Pure gonadoblastoma varies in size from a small histological lesion to about 8 cm mass. Much larger tumors occur, if gonadoblastoma is overgrown by dysgerminoma/seminoma or other germ cell tumors. The appearance of sectioned mass is influenced by the presence of hyalinization, calcification or amount of overgrown germ cell tumor.

Microscopic

Gonadoblastoma is a tumor composed of two main cell types, germ cells, which are similar to those of dysgerminoma/seminoma and sex cord derivatives resembling immature Sertoli or granulosa cells. The tumor has a characteristic pattern of cellular tubular islands of intimately mixed germ cells and sex cord mesenchymal cells (Figure 39 A, B, C). The germ cells are large with often clear cytoplasm and large vesicular nuclei with prominent nucleoli. Mitotic activity may be present. The immature Sertoli and granulosa cells are smaller and epithelial like. These cells are arranged in coronal pattern along the periphery of the nests, surrounding single or groups of germ cells or surrounding small round spaces containing eosinophilic PAS positive material resembling Call Exner bodies.

In the clinicopathologic analysis of 74 cases of gonadoblastoma, Scully 142 observed that foci of calcification replaced the tumor cells and the surrounding stroma became fibrosed and hyalinized. This resulted into the formation of fibro calcific masses in which viable tumor cells were rather sparse or absent. On gross examination, 33 out of 74 cases (44%) revealed calcification and in 17 cases calcification was identified on roentgenogram of pelvis. Figure 39 D is from a case of gonadoblastoma showing scattered germ cells intimately mixed with sex cord mesenchymal cells, note conspicuous focal calcification. No superimposed dysgerminoma or any other malignant germ cell tumor was present.

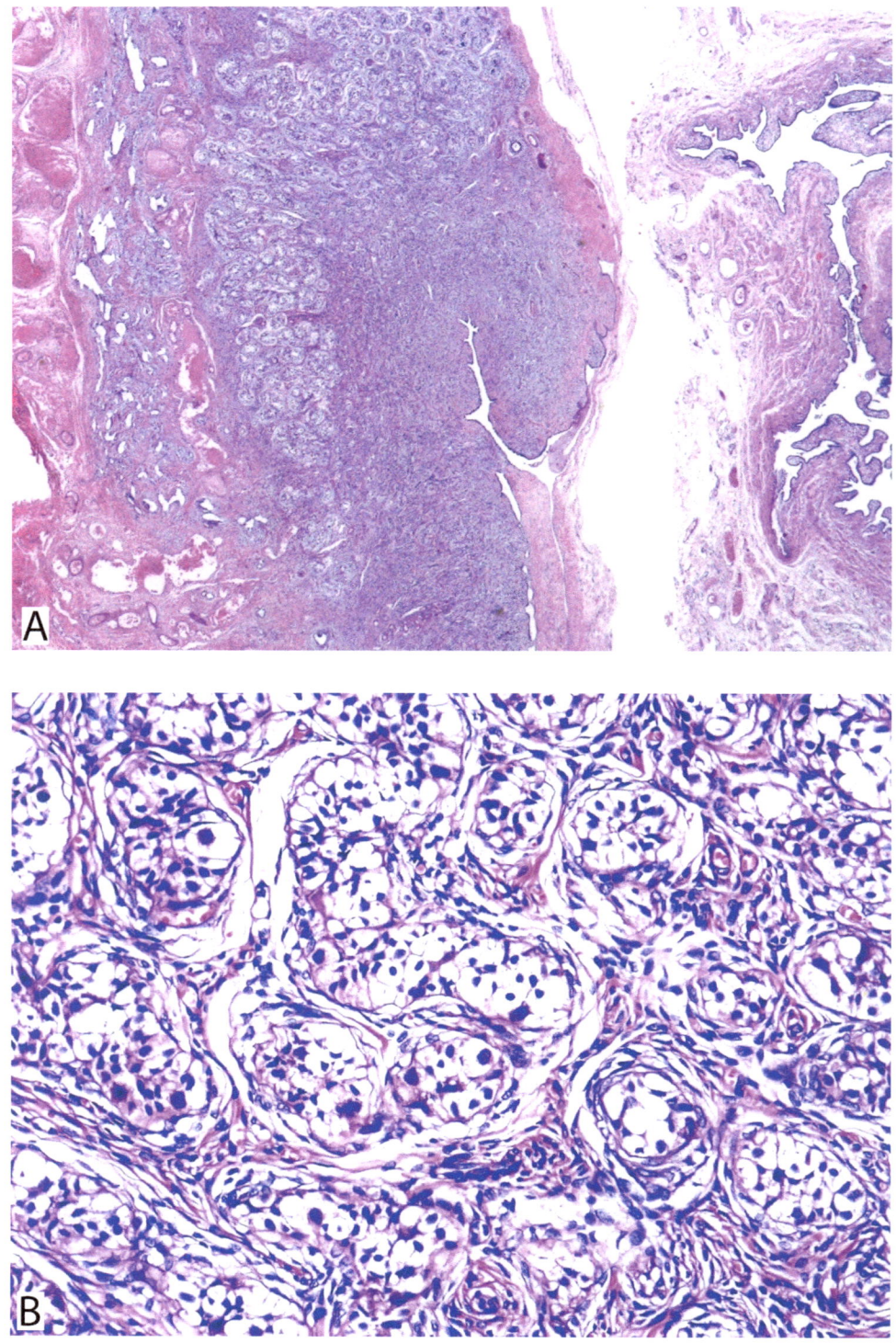

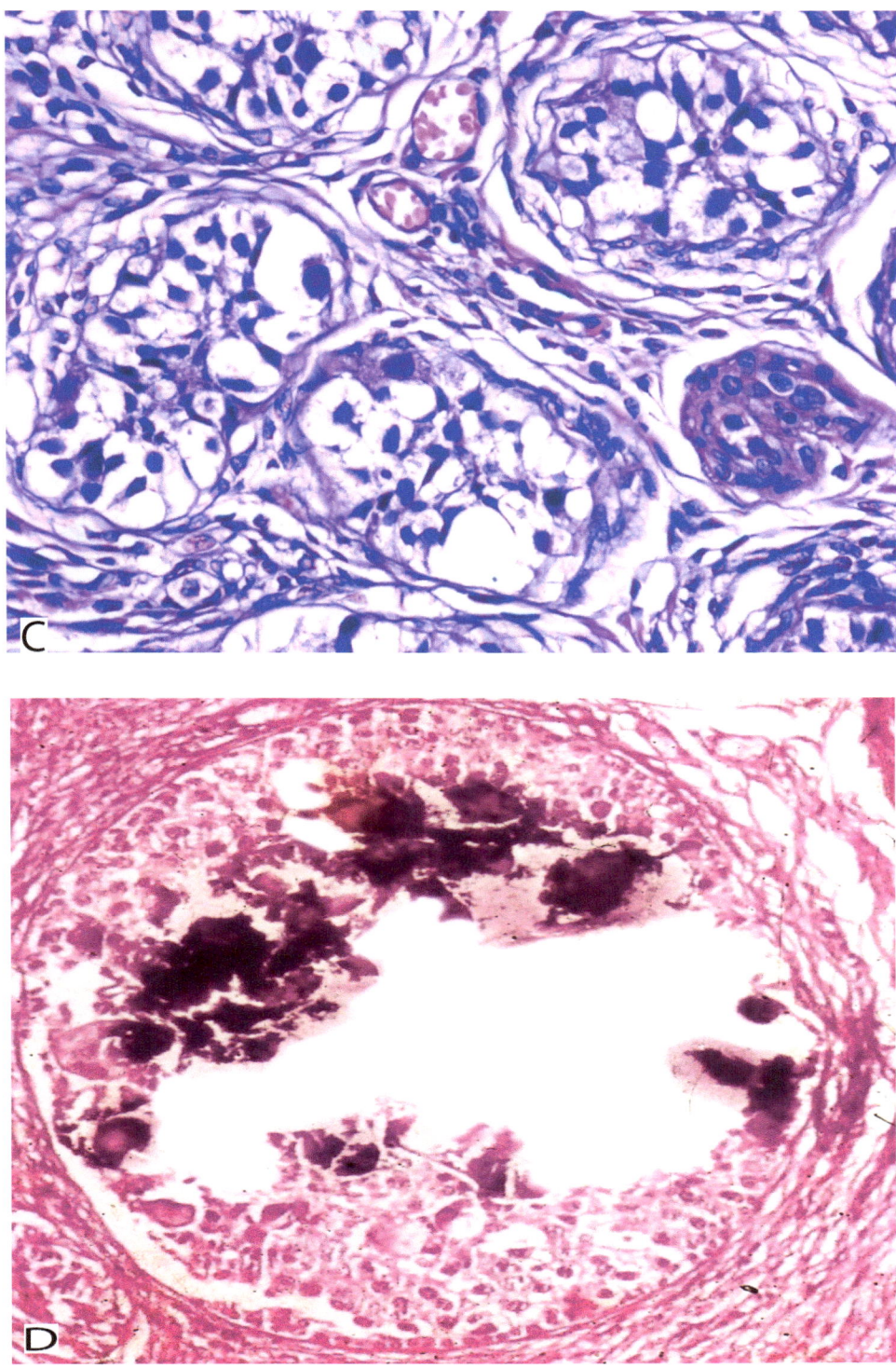

Figure 39 (A) Scanner view shows a streak dysgenetic gonad (Ovary) covered with a solid sheet of gonadoblastoma tubules (B) low power showing few larger cell (germ cells) (arrow heads)and sex cord cells (C)high power view We are indebted to Dr Jay Mehta Oncopathologist SRL Ranbaxy Mumbai for this Figure (D)Another case: The oval cell mass shows diffuse degenerative changes and blotches of dystrophic calcification, few scattered germ cells each within large vacuole and surrounding sex cord cells seen; a phenotypically female with infertility had dysgenetic gonad with a 1.5 cm circumscribed nodule

Prognosis

Patients having gonadoblastoma with malignant germ cell tumor are treated by surgical excision of the gonads without additional treatment. The patients with superimposed malignant germ cell tumor are treated with surgery and chemotherapy; the latter is quite effective. It has been observed that dysgerminoma arising in gonadoblastoma tends to metastasize less frequently and at a later stage than dysgerminoma arising de novo 142.

The importance of gonadoblastoma, in addition to its association with intersex conditions, is its propensity to give rise to malignant germ cell tumors, particularly dysgerminoma/seminoma 143, 144.

Metastatic Tumors in ovaries ("Krukenberg tumors")

Definition

A bilaterally occurring metastatic tumor of mucin producing epithelial cells is usually derived from a primary gastrointestinal mucinous adenocarcinoma. Histologically it has been defined as an ovarian carcinoma that contains a significant component of mucin filled signet ring cells, typically lying within a cellular stroma of spindly cells (Figure 40 A-D)

Ovary is a relatively frequent site for metastatic carcinomas from various organs, especially stomach, colon, breast and pancreas. In 1896, Friedrich Krukenberg described 6 cases of bilateral ovarian tumors and published them as fibrosarcoma ovarii mucocellulare (carcinomatodes). He observed a typical signet ring carcinomatous growth accompanied by a striking spindle cell proliferation, which he interpreted as fibrosarcoma. He believed that these were primary ovarian tumors 145. Over the years, several studies have proved that some clinically apparent primary ovarian tumors represent metastases from primary in other organs in the body especially gastrointestinal tract (Figure 40), pancreas 146, gall bladder/biliary tract 147, cervix 148 etc.; 10% of all ovarian tumors are metastatic carcinomas. Rarely, the metastasis may precede detection of the primary sites and may present as an ovarian tumor. In a study of 147 patients with ovarian metastases from extragenital primary cancer, following site wise distribution was recorded: colorectal region (49%), gastric (40.8%), breast (8.2%), biliary tract (1.4%), and liver (0.7%) 149.

Distinction between Primary and Metastatic Mucinous Carcinomas of the Ovary

Among ovarian epithelial tumors the mucinous tumors pose the greatest difficulty with regard to distinction of primary from metastatic ovarian tumors. Tumors that have mucinous cell type offer a particular challenge; description of primary mucinous ovarian tumors in the earlier literature often included some tumors that were actually metastatic 150. This dilemma has prompted a number of recent studies, which have clarified the morphologic findings of primary mucinous carcinoma 151, 152, 153.

The literature concerning metastatic ovarian carcinomas is focused on primary tumors from specific sites that have spread to the ovaries with associated problems, and role of immunohistochemistry in primary versus metastatic mucinous ovarian cancers. The primary ovarian mucinous tumors (borderline mucinous and carcinomas) can be usually easily separated from metastatic mucinous ovarian carcinomas on the basis of a thorough morphological analysis 150.

Primary Mucinous; Diagnostic criteria:

Typically large (>15 cm) in size
Smooth capsular surface
Usually unassociated with extra ovarian disease
Complex papillary pattern
Benign or borderline areas (microscopically)
Expansile growth pattern

Secondary mucinous: Diagnostic criteria

Bilaterality
Surface involvement by carcinoma cells
Microscopic surface mucin
Infiltrative pattern of stromal invasion
Ovarian hilar involvement
Vascular invasion

Microscopic: Immunohistochemistry

Despite studies providing refined morphologic diagnostic criteria for ovarian mucinous tumors, the problem of distinguishing primary from metastatic persists. To unravel this problem ancillary studies using immunohistochemical evaluation have been carried out and reported in many review articles 154, 155, 156, 157, 158. Coordinate Immunophenotypes of CK7 +ve/ CK20 –ve and CK7 +ve/CK20 +ve can usually separate tumors of upper GI tract from those of lower GI tract (recto sigmoid and appendiceal) 10. The latter express CK7 –ve/CK20 +ve immunophenotype. Both primary and secondary mucinous tumors may show overlapping immunophenotype expression. Hence, prediction of likely primary site is best accomplished by combined analysis of morphologic features and a panel of markers 10

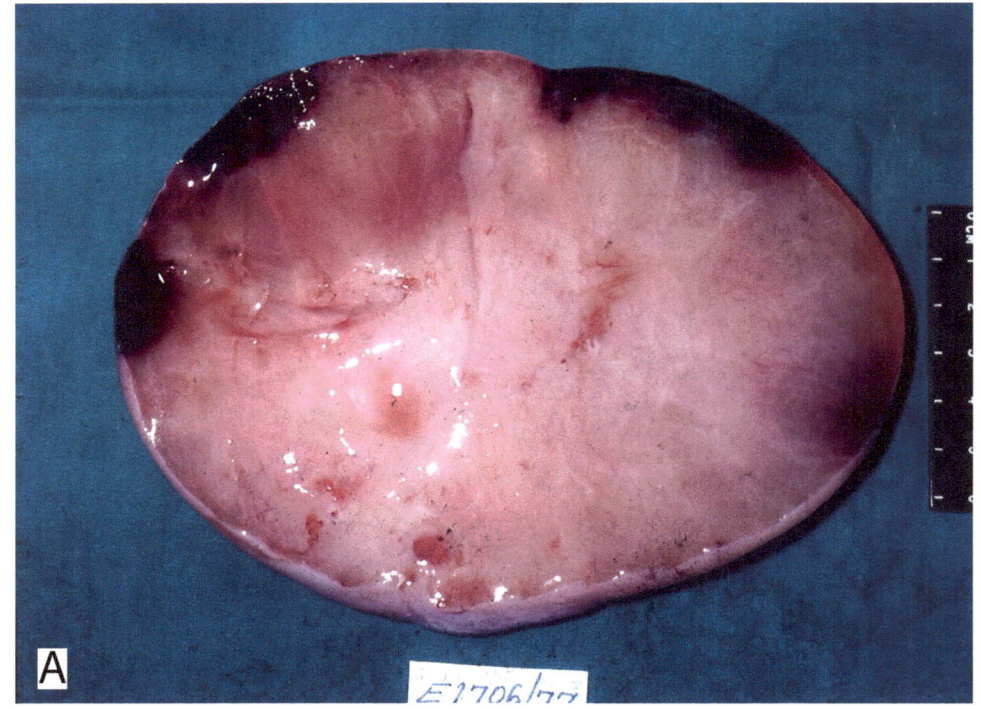
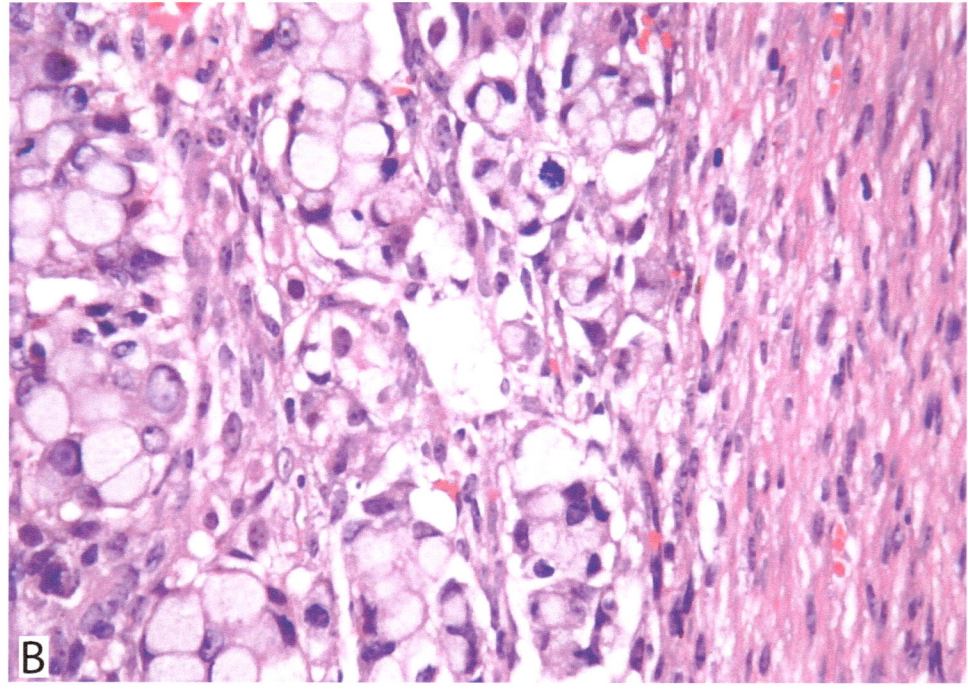

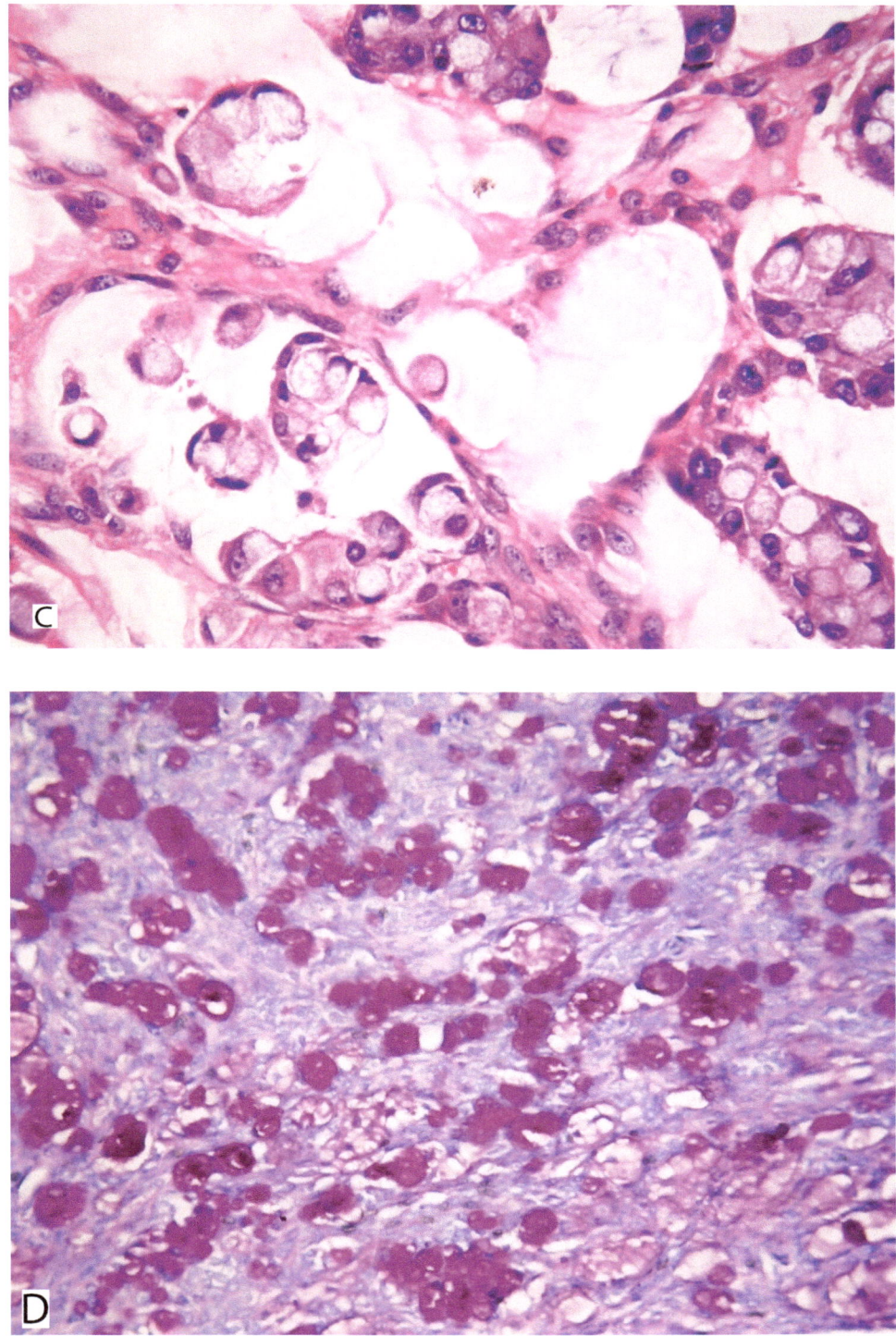

Figure 40 'Krukenberg tumor' (A) tumor bearing ovary shows soft grey slightly translucent gelatinous tissue with focal hemorrhages foci; (B, C) singles and small groups of mucin filled signet ring cells and variable intervening stroma; (D) Signet ring cells filled with PAS positive mucin. A 45 year woman had bilateral ovarian masses, upon investigations a signet ring cell adenocarcinoma(biopsy proven) was detected in stomach

DIAGNOSTIC PROBLEMS IN TUMORS OF FEMALE GENITAL TRACT: SELECTED TOPICS

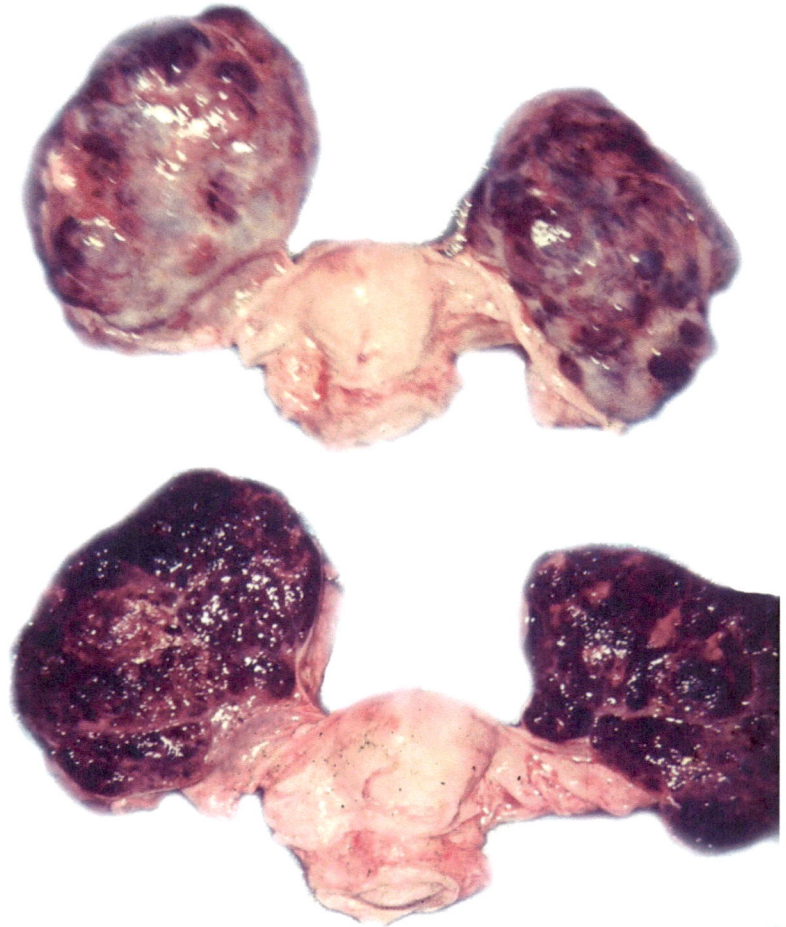

Figure 41, HIV positive woman having primary angiosarcoma of breast with metastases to both ovaries (detected at autopsy); according to the definition the term Krukenberg tumor is inappropriate in this case.

Aggressive Angiomyxoma (AAM)

Definition

The term aggressive angiomyxoma (now designated as deep angiomyxoma by WHO) ,was coined by Steerper and Rosai in 1983 159 for a morphologically distinctive slow growing neoplasm occurring in the genital, perianal and pelvic regions of adult females. It is histologically bland but known to recur in large proportion of cases.

Clinical findings

The patients present with a relatively large often greater than 10 cm, slowly growing, painless mass in the pelvi-perineal region. Clinical misdiagnosis, most common as Bartholin's cyst, is a common finding in as many as 82% of cases. This rare tumor occurs almost exclusively in females, the male to female ratio being 1:6 in favor of females. In males the AAM has been described in scrotum, inguinal region, spermatic cord and pelvis. The tumor is quite rare and in a period of 26 years [1983 to 2009] only 100 cases have been reported worldwide (including 24 males) 159, 160, 161, 162, 163.

Gross

The tumor is soft, circumscribed or polypoid, gelatinous on cut surface and range in size from few cm to 20 cm or even more (Figure 42 A, B) Although it is often sharply defined in some areas, it presents adhesions or infiltration in the surrounding soft tissues.

Microscopic

Short spindle and stellate shaped cells are evenly spread out in an abundant myxoid stroma and there are haphazardly scattered small and large blood vessels, some having hypertrophy or hyalinization of the wall . The nuclear morphology is totally bland and pathologist unfamiliar with this tumor will believe that it is benign (Figure 42 C-D). However, the lesion is deceptively benign and the reported recurrence rate varies from 35% to 72%, even with clear surgical margins 164.

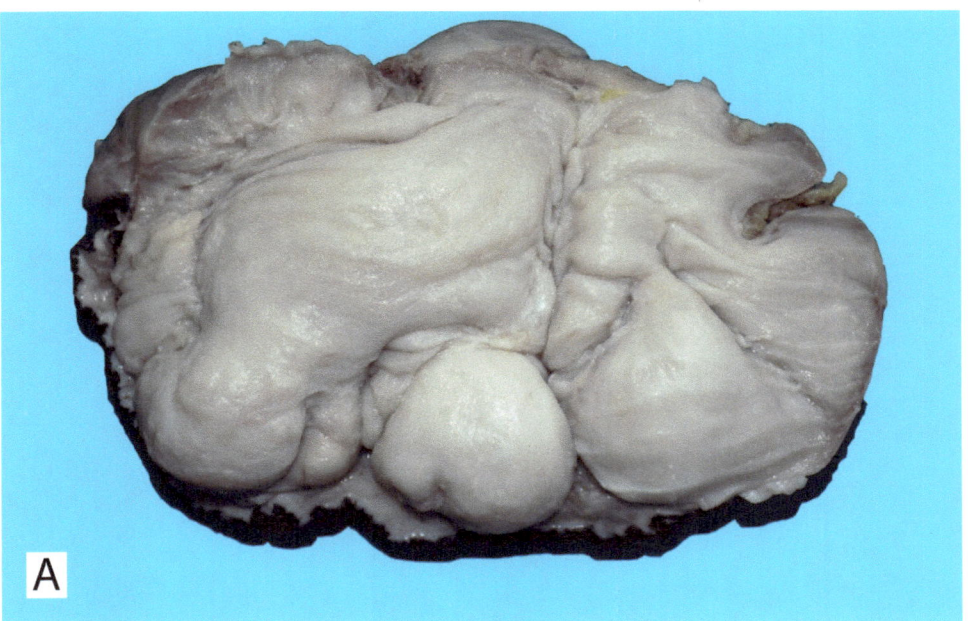

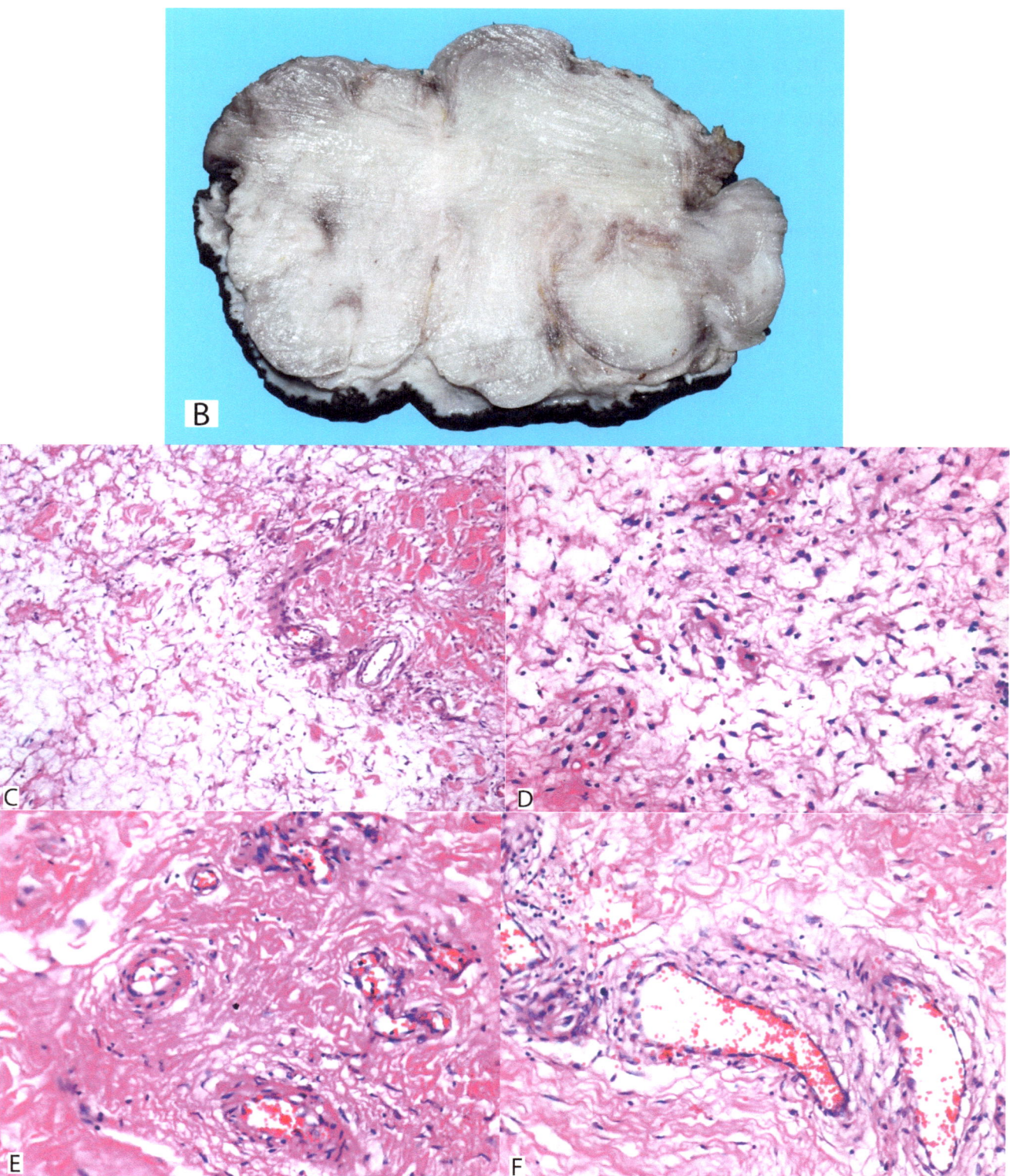

Figure 42 Aggressive angiomyxoma. Recurrent tumor of Vulva- size 14 x 12 x 6 cm) (A &B) large, well defined lobular, grey white soft tissue mass sharply defined from vulvar skin (lower border); (C&D) close up of myxomatous element; sparse cellularity (E&F) Large number of vessels of variable calibers, thick walled vessels and lack of nuclear atypia are defining features of this tumor.

Immunophenotype

Immunohistochemically the stromal cells consistently stain for vimentin and variably for muscle specific actin, but not for smooth muscle actin, desmin and S-100. Many previous reports have demonstrated estrogen and progesterone receptor positivity in this neoplasm. Five cases of aggressive angiomyxoma in female patients and one involving male pelvic soft parts were stained for antibodies to ER and PR, in one series. All females showed variable positivity to ER and PR but was not detected in the single male patient in this study. Dermal fibroblasts, normal vulvar skin and stromal cells in a variety of vulvar lesions have also been found to be positive for ER and PR. Therefore this test can-not be used to distinguish aggressive angiomyxoma and its histological mimics.

It is of interest to know that ER and PR positivity has also been observed in fibromatosis and there have been reports of a dramatic clinical response to the antiestrogen tamoxifen in some cases. The estrogen and progesterone receptor positivity suggests that AAM might be hormone dependent, as rapid growth has been observed during pregnancy165, 166.

Differential Diagnosis

Aggressive angiomyxoma should be differentiated from myxoid liposarcoma, myxoid fibrosarcoma etc., which have metastatic potential. The tumor has a local recurrence rate of approximately 30%, and such recurrences are usually controlled by a single re-excision. Thus, this tumor is less aggressive than was originally believed and has no known metastatic potential 167.

PEComa of the Female Genital Tract

Perivascular epithelioid cell tumor (PEComa) refers to a family of tumors, which are defined by their co-expression of melanocytic (HMB-45, S100 & Melan A) and muscle (SMA, Desmin) markers. The currently reported PEComas include renal and extra-renal angiomyolipoma, lymphangioleiomyomatosis, clear cell "sugar" tumor of the lung, clear cell myomelanocytic tumors of the falciform ligament/ligamentum teres and distinctive clear cell tumors at other anatomical sites 168, 169.

The uterus is the most prevalent reported site of involvement of PEComa-not otherwise specified (NOS). In one report on PEComa of uterus (2007), there were 38 cases of uterine involvement among 100 PEComas (NOS). All three lesions in this case showed identical histology of biphasic growth pattern of transition from spindle cells and epithelioid cells (Figure 43 A-C), often arranged around vascular spaces. The tumor cells express melanocytic markers (Figure 43 D). The literature review indicated that PEComa-NOS are tumors of uncertain malignant potential, and metastases to other organs might become evident even several years after primary diagnosis 170.

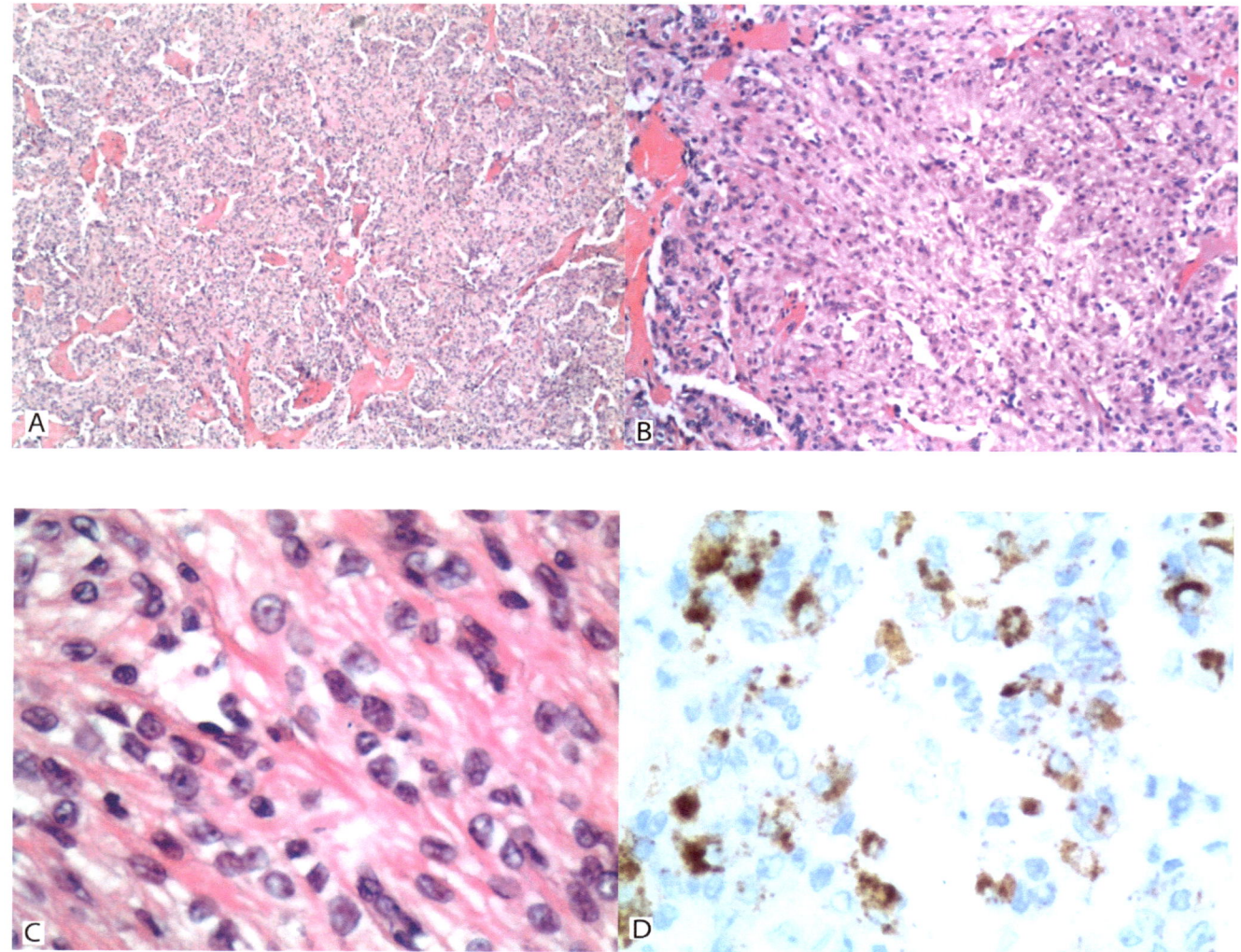

Figure 43 (A) Groups and sheets of mainly "epithelioid" cells traversed by thick hyaline bands; (B) epithelioid cells with pale staining or vacuolated cytoplasm (C) a mixture of spindly cell with eosinophilic cells and sparsely populated vacuolated or clear cells (D) HMB 45 is expressed as abundant granular brownish pigment in the cytoplasm

Fallopian Tube Serous Carcinoma &Molecular Pathogenesis of Ovarian Carcinoma

Ovarian carcinoma was traditionally thought to originate from the ovarian surface epithelium or ovarian epithelial inclusions, and investigative efforts at early detection have been centered on the ovary for decades. However, these efforts have not been successful and the overall dismal survival for women with ovarian cancer has not changed over the last 50 years. The recent morphologic and molecular genetic studies have led to a paradigm shift in our concepts of the carcinogenesis and histogenesis of ovarian and peritoneal serous carcinomas. In 2001, a group of Dutch investigators 171 showed dysplastic lesions in prophylactically removed fallopian tubes of women predisposed to developing ovarian cancer. The dysplastic changes resembled histology of high grade serous ovarian carcinoma and now several studies have endorsed the theory that origin of tubal and ovarian serous carcinomas is in the precursor lesion of the tubal mucosa.

It has been found that as many as 30% of patients with fallopian tube carcinoma have germline BRCA1 or BRCA2 mutations 172, 173 Studies of step-serial transverse sections from tubes (including fimbriae) of women with BRCA mutations or family history of breast or ovarian cancer resulted in detection of early tubal serous carcinoma or small invasive serous carcinoma in 2.5% to17% of patients 174, 175. Many serous carcinomas presumed to be of ovarian or peritoneal origin are associated with serous tubal intraepithelial carcinoma, which is evidently a precursor lesion in fallopian tube mucosa 176.Women with BRCA mutations carry a significant risk of pelvic serous carcinoma that reaches as high as 60%, if followed indefinitely.

Microscopic

In a clinicopathologic study of 105 cases of carcinoma of fallopian tube 177, 50% were serous, 25% endometrioid, 11% transitional, 8% undifferentiated, 4% mixed type, and 2% clear cell type. Serous carcinoma of the fallopian tube is the most common type (50%) with a very aggressive behavior. The histological features will be described at length.

The serous tubal intraepithelial carcinomas (STIC) detected in risk-reducing salpingo-oophorectomy specimens are typically microscopic (< 1-2 mm) and usually occur in the fimbriae and distal tube. The characteristic features include loss of ciliated cells, epithelial and nuclear stratification, nuclear enlargement with high N/C ratio, prominent nucleoli, loss of polarity and presence of mitotic activity (Figure 44 A, B, C) 178. Immunohistochemical stains help confirm the diagnosis and increase diagnostic reproducibility. STICs display strong and diffuse immunostaining for p53and a high proliferation index with Ki 67 (Figure D, E)

Fallopian tubes from women with and without BRCA mutations have recently been found to contain clusters of epithelial cells with immunostaining for p53, called p53 signatures 172, 174. The signature lesion has been defined as a stretch of at least 12 morphologically benignp53 positive secretory cells with a low proliferative (ki67) index. The p53 signature lesion is a finding that has been proposed to be a nonmalignant potential precursor lesion to serous tubal in situ carcinoma179, 180.

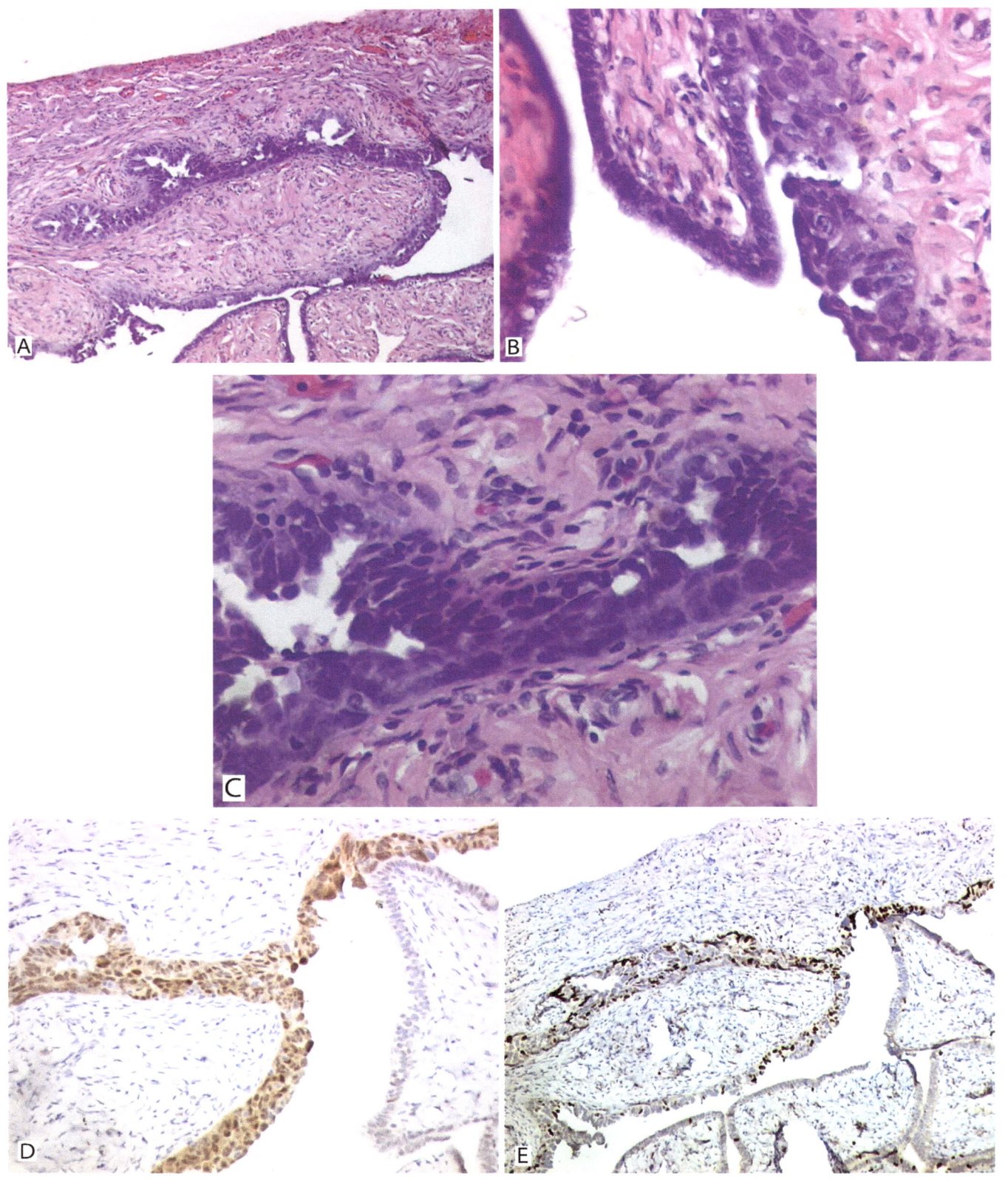

Figure 44 (A, B, C) Low and high power views of Carcinoma in situ of follopian tube; (D) diffuse and strong nuclear positivity with p53 immunostain; (E) neoplastic epithelial cells express Ki 67

References

Endometrial Hyperplasia

1) Scully RE, BonFigurelio TA, Kurman RJ, et al. Uterine corpus. In: World Health Organization: Histological typing of Female Genital Tract Tumors, 1994 Springer-Verlag: New York, pp 13-31

2) Lidor A, Ismajovich B, Confino E, et al. Histopathological findings in 226 women with postmenopausal uterine bleeding. Acta Obstet Gynecol Scand 1986; 65:-41-43

3) Mazur MT. Endometrial hyperplasia/adenocarcinoma A conventional approach Ann DignPathol 2005; 9:174-181

4) Horn LC, Schnurrbusch U, Bilek K, et al. Risk of progression in complex and atypical endometrial hyperplasia: clinicopathologic analysis in cases with and without progestogen treatment. Int J Gynecol Cancer 2004; 14:348-353

5) Kendall HD, Ronnett BM, Isacson C, et al. Reproducibility of the diagnosis endometrial hyperplasia, atypical hyperplasia and well differentiated adenocarcinoma. Am J SurgPathol 1998; 22:1012-1029

6) Bergeron C, Nogales FF, Masseroli M, et al. A multicentric European study testing the reproducibility of the WHO classification of endometrial hyperplasia with a proposal of a simplified working classification for biopsy and curettage specimens Am J SurgPathol 1999; 23:1102-1108

7) Silverberg SG, Kurman RJ, Nogales F, et al. Tumors of the uterine Corpus In: Tavassoli FA, Deville P. editors Pathology and genetics of the tumours of the breast and female genital organs. World Health Organization classification of tumours, Lyon, France: IARC Press; 2003 p 217-232

8) Kurman RJ, Kaminski PF, Norris HJ. The behavior of endometrial hyperplasia: A long term study of "untreated" hyperplasia in 170 patients. Cancer 1985; 56:403-412

9) Horn LC, Meinel A, Handzel R et al Histopathology of endometrial hyperplasia and endometrial carcinoma: An Update. Ann DignPathol 2007; 11: 297-311

Endometrioid Adenocarcinoma with Squamous Differentiation

10) Zaino RJ, Kurman RJ, Herbold D, et al. The significance of Squamous Differentiation in Endometrial Carcinoma. Cancer 1991; 68:2293-2302

11) Haqqani MT, Fox H. Adenosquamous carcinoma of the endometrium. J ClinPathol 1976; 29:959-966

12) Aneler VM, Kjorstad KE. Endometrial Adenocarcinoma with Squamous Cell Differentiation. Cancer1992:69:488-495

13) Zaino RJ, Kurman RJ. Squamous differentiation in carcinoma of the endometrium: a critical appraisal of adenoacanthoma and adenosquamous carcinoma. SeminDiagnPathol 1988; 5:154-171

Endometrial Serous papillary carcinoma

14) Gitsch G, Friedlander ML, Wain GV, et al. Uterine Papillary Serous Carcinoma: A Clinical Study Cancer 1995; 75:2239-2243

15 Abelar VM, Kjorstad KE. Endometrial carcinoma in Norway: A study of total population. Cancer 1991; 67: 3093-3103

16) Hendrickson M, MartinezA, Ross J, et al. Uterine papillary serous carcinoma: A highly malignant form of endometrial adenocarcinoma. Am J SurgPathol 1982; 6:93-108

17 Darvishian F, Hummer AJ, Thaler HT, et al. Serous Endometrial Cancers That Mimic Endometrioid Adenocarcinoma: A Clinicopathologic and Immunohistochemical Study of a Group of Problematic Cases. Am J SurgPathol 2004; 28:1568-1578 5

18) Wheelar DT, Bell KA, Kurman RJ, et al. Minimal uterine serous carcinoma: Diagnosis and clinicopathologic correlation. Am J SurgPathol 2000; 24:797-806

19) Soslow RA; Pirog E, Isacson C. Endometrial Intraepithelial Carcinoma with Associated Peritoneal Carcinomatosis. Am J SurgPathol 2000; 24:726-732

20) Trehan S, Tetu B, Raymond PE. Serous papillary carcinoma of the endometrium arising from endometrial polyps: a clinical, histological and immunohistochemical study of 13 cases. Human Pathol 2005; 36:1316-1321

21) Abeler VM, Kjordstad K, Berle E. Carcinoma of endometrium in Norway: a histopathologic and prognostic survey of a total population. Int J Gynecol Cancer1992; 2:9-22

Clear Cell Endometrial Carcinoma

22) Kurman RJ, Scully RE. Clear Cell Carcinoma of the Endometrium: An Analysis of 21 cases. Cancer 1976; 37:872-882

23) Fadare O, Liang SX, Ulukus EC, et al. Precursors of endometrial clear cell carcinoma. Am J Surg Pathol 2006; 30:1519-1530

24) Abeler VM, Vergote RB, Kjorstad KE, et al. Clear Cell Carcinoma of the Endometrium: Prognosis and Metastatic Pattern.

25) Fadare O, Zheng W, Crispens MA. Morphological and other clinicopathologic features of endometrial clear cell carcinoma: a comprehensive analysis of 50 rigorously classified cases. Am J Cancer Res 2013; 3:70-95

Endometrial Adenocarcinoma in Infertile women

26) Fadhlaoui A, Hassouna JB, Krouf M, et al. Endometrial Adenocarcinoma in a 27 year old Woman. Clinical Medicine Insights: Case Reports 2010; 3:31-39

27) Beliere M, Radikof G, Galant C, et al. Identification of women at high risk of developing endometrial cancer on tamoxiphen. Eur j Cancer 2000; 36:35-36

28) Vaccarello L, Apte SM, Copeland LJ, et al. Endometrial adenocarcinoma associated pregnancy; a report of three cases and a literature review GynecolOncol 1999; 74: 118-122

29) Kim YB, Holschneider CH, Ghosh K, et al Progestin Alone as Primary Treatment of Endometrial Carcinoma in Premenopausal Women: Report of Cases and Review of the Literature. Cancer 1997; 79:320-327

30) Chiva L, Lapuente L, Gonzales-Cortija L, et al. Sparing fertility in young women with endometrial cancer.GynecolOncol 2008; 111:101-104

31) Wang CB, Wang CJ, Huang HJ. Fertility Preserving Treatment in Young Patients with Endometrial adenocarcinoma Cancer 2002; 94:2192-2198

Malignant Mixed Mullerian Tumor (MMMT)

32) Kanthan R, Senger JL. Review Article Uterine carcinomas (Malignant Mixed Mullerian Tumors): A review with Special Emphasis on the Controversies in Management. Obstetrics and Gynecology International 2011; Article ID 470795

33)) El-Nashar SA, Mariani A. "Uterine Carcinosarcoma" Clinical Obstetrics and Gynecology 2011; 54: 292-304

34) Abell MR, Ramirez JA. Sarcomas and carcinosarcomas of the uterine cervix Cancer 1973; 31:1176-1192

35) George E, Manivel JC, Dehner LP, et al. Malignant mixed Mullerian tumors: An immunohistochemical study of 47 cases, with histogenetic considerations and clinical correlation. Hum Pathol 1991; 22: 215-223

36) Amant E, Moreman P, Davel GH, et al. Uterine carcinosarcoma with melanocytic differentiation. Int J GynecolPathol, 2001; 20:186-190

37) Shokeir MO, Noel SM, Clement PB. Malignant Mullerian Mixed Tumor of the Uterus with a prominent alpha-fetoprotein producing component of yolk sac tumor Mod Pathol 1996; 9:647-651

38) Bitterman P, Chun B, Kurman RJ. The Significance of Epithelial Differentiation in Mixed Mesodermal Tumors of the Uterus: A clinicopathologic and Immunohistochemical Study. Am J SurgPathol 1990; 14:317-328

39) Ferguson SE, Tornos C, Hummer A, et al. Prognostic features of surgical stage I uterine carcinosarcoma. Am J SurgPathol 2007; 31:1653-1661

REFERENCES

Mullerian Adenosarcoma

40) Clement PB, Scully RE. Mullerian adenosarcoma of uterus: a clinicopathologic analysis of 10 cases of a distinctive type of Mullerian mixed tumor Cancer 1974; 341138-1149

41) Clement PB, Scully RE. Mullerian adenosarcoma of the uterus: a clinicopathologic analysis of 100 cases with a review of the literature. Hum Pathol 1990; 21:363-381

42) Clement PB. Mullerian sarcoma of the uterus with sarcomatous overgrowth: a clinicopathologic analysis of 10 cases Am J SurgPathol 1989; 113:28-38

43) Gallardo A, Prat J. Mullerian Adenosarcoma: A clinicopathologic and Immunohistochemical Study of 55 Cases Challenging the Existence of Adenofibroma. Am J SurgPathol 2009; 33:278-288

44) Soslow RA, AlliAsya, Olivia E. Mullerian Adenosarcoma: An immunophenotypic analysis of 35 cases. Am J SurgPathol 2008; 32:1013-1021

45) Mikami Y, Hata S, C.T., Kiyokawa T, et al. Expression of CD10 In Malignant Mullerian Mixed Tumors and Adenosarcomas: An Immunohistochemical Study. Mod Pathol 2001; 15:923-930

Endometrial Stromal Sarcoma (ESS)

46) Puliath G, Nair K. Endometrial stromal sarcoma: A review of the Literature. Indian J Med PaediatOncol 2012; 33:1-6

47) Kurihara S, Oda Y, Ohishi Y, et al.Endometrial Stromal Sarcoma and Related High-grade Sarcomas: Immunohistochemical Molecular Genetic Study of 31 Cases. Am J SurgPathol 2008:32:1248-1238

48) Aubry M-C, Myers JL, Colby TV, et al. Endometrial Stromal Sarcoma Metastatic to the Lung. Am J Surg Pathol 2002; 26; 440-449

49) Ramia JM, Plaza R, Garcia R, et al. Liver metastasis of endometrial stromal sarcoma. World J Hepatol 2012; 4:415-418

50) Gabel S, Ashour Z, Hamada G, et al Low Grade Endometrial Sarcoma with Intravenous Extension to the Heart. Medscape J Med 2009; 11:23:1-5

51) Chu PG, Arber DA, Weiss LM, et all. Utility of CD10 in distinguishing between endometrial stromal sarcoma and uterine smooth muscle tumors: An immunohistochemical comparison of 34 cases. Mod Pathol 2001; 14:465—471

Leiomyosarcoma of Uterus

52) Hendrickson MR, Tavassoli FA, Kempson RL, et al. Mesenchymal tumor and related lesions. In Tavassoli FA, Deville P (Ed)Pathology and Genetics.Tumors of the Breast and Female Genital Organs. Edited by WHO Classification of Tumors, IARC Press, Lyon 2003,pp 236

53)Harlow BL, Weiss NS, Lofton S. The epidemiology of the sarcomas of the uterus. J Natl Can Inst 1986;76:399-402

54) Leibsohn S, D'ablaing G, Mishell DR Jr et al. Lieomyosarcoma in a series of hysterectomies performed for a presumed uterine leiomyoma. Am J ObstGynecol 1990;162:968-974

55)Nucci MR. Tumors of the Female Genital Tract, Part D- Myometrium.In Fletcher CDM.Diagnostic Histopathology of TumorsVol 1, Fourth Ed. Elsevier Saunders 2013.

56) Bell SW, Kempson RL, Hendrickson MR. Problematic Uterine smooth muscle neoplasms. A clinicopathologic studyof 213 cases.Am J SurgPathol 1994;18:535-558

56 a) Philip PC, Annie N.Y. Cheung, Clement PB. Uterine Smooth Muscle Tumors of Uncertain Malignant Potential (STUMP) Am J SurgPathol 2009; 33:99201005

57) Downes KA, Hart WR. Bizarre Leiomyomas of the Uterus: A Comprehensive Pathologic study of 24 cases With long- term follow- up Am J SurgPathol 1997;21:1261-7058)

58) Prayson RA, Goldblum JR, Hart WR. Epithelioid smooth muscle tumors of the uterus: A clinicopathologic study of 18 cases Am J Surg Pathol1997; 21:383-391

Minimal deviation adenocarcinoma

59) Silverberg SG, Hurt WG. Minimal deviation adenocarcinoma ("adenoma malignum") of the cervix: a reappraisal. Am J ObstetGynecol 1975; 121:971-975

60) Kaminsky PF, Norris HJ. Minimal deviation of adenocarcinoma (adenoma malignum) of the cervix, Int j GynecolPathol 1983; 2:141-152

61) Pirog EC, Kleter B. Et al. Prevalence of human papilloma virus DNA in different histological subtypes of cervical adenocarcinoma. Am J Pathol 2000; 157:1055-1062

62) Young RH, Welch WR, et al. Ovarian sex cord tumor with annular tubules: a review of 74 cases including 27 with PeutzJeghers syndrome and 4 with adenoma malignum of the cervix. Cancer 1982; 50:1384-1402

63) Gilks CB, Young RH, Aguirre P, et al. Adenoma Malignum (Minimal Deviation Adenocarcinoma) of the Uterine Cervix: A clinicopathologic and Immunohistochemical Analysis of 26 cases. Am J SurgPathol 1989; 13:717-729

64) Gong Li, Zhang WD, Liu XY Clinical status and clinicopathologic observation of cervical minimal deviation adenocarcinoma. Diagnostic Pathology 2010; 5:25

Glandular Lesions of Cervix Mimicking Cancer & Cervical Glandular Intraepithelial Neoplasia (CGIN)

65) McCluggage WG Glandular lesions of the uterine cervix . Current Diagnostic Pathology 2000, 6,

66) Leminen A, Paavonen J, Forss M et al. Adenocarcinoma of the uterine cervix
Cancer 1990;65:53-59

67) Grayson W, Cooper K. Application of immunohistochemistry in the evaluation of neoplastic epithelial lesions of the uterine cervix and endometrium. Current Diagnostic Pathology 2003,9, 19-25

68) McCluggageWG Metaplasia in the female genital tract. Recent Advances in Histopathology Vol.20.Edited by David Lowe, James Underwood. The Royal Society of Medicine Press Ltd. 2003

69) Mikami Y. McCluggage WG. Endocervical glandular lesions exhibiting gastric differentiation: an emerging spectrum of benign, premalignant, and malignant lesions AdvaAnatPathol 2013 Jul;20(4):227-37. doi: 10.1097/PAP.0b013e31829c2d66

70) Kawakami F, Mikami Y, Kojima A, Ito M, Nishimura R, Manabe T. Diagnostic reproducibility in gastric-type mucinous adenocarcinoma of the uterine cervix: validation of novel diagnostic criteria. Histopathology 2010 Mar;56(4):551-3. doi: 10.1111/j.1365-2559.2010.03500.x.

71) Medeiros F, Bell DA. Pseudoneoplastic lesions of the female genital tract Arch path Lab Med 2010;134:393-

72) Park KJ, Soslow RA. Current concepts in cervical pathology. Arch Path Lab med 2009;133:729-38

73) Anagnostopoulos A, Ruthven S, Kingston R. Mesonephric adenocarcinoma of the uterine cervix and literature review. BMJ Case Rep 2012;Dec 10;2012

74) McClugggae WG. New developments in endocervical glandular lesions. Histopathology 2013;62:136-60

75) Shukla A, Thomas D, Roh MH. PAX8 and PAX2 expression in endocervical adenocarionoma in situ and high grade squamous dysplasia. Int J Gynecol Pathol 2013;32:116-21

Melanoma of Female Genital Tract

76)) Change AE, Kamell LH, ,Menck HR. The national cancer data base report on cutaneous and noncutaneous melanoma: A summary o 84, 836 cases from the past decade. Cancer 1998; 83:1663-1678

77) Giuliano AE, Cohran AJ, Morton DL. Melanoma from unknown primary site and amelanotic melanoma.Semin Oncol1982; 9:442-447

78) Duggal R, Shrinivason R. Primary amelanotic melanoma of the cervix: case report with review of literature. J gynecolOncol 2010; Vol 21: 199-202

79) McLaughlin CC, Wu XC, Jemal A, et al. Incidence of noncutaneous melanomas in the U.S. Cancer 2005; 103:1000-1007

80) Seetharamu N, Ott PA, Palick AC. Mucosal Melanomas: A Case-Based Review of the Literature. The Oncologist 2010; 15:772-781

81) Ragnarson-Olding BK, Kanter-Lewensohn LR, Lagerlof B, et al Malignant Melanoma of the Vulva in a Nationwide 25-Year Study of 219 Swedish Females. Cancer 1999; 86:1273-1284

82) Ragnarson-Olding BK, Johansson H, Rutquist L-E. Et al. Malignant Melanoma of the Vulva and Vagina: Trends in Incidence, Age Distribution, and Long-term Survival among 245 Consecutive Cases in Sweden 1960-1984. Cancer 1993; 71: 1893-1897

83) Preti M, Micheletti L, Massobrio M, et al. Vulvar Paget's disease: one century after first reported. J Low Genit Tract Dis 2003;7:122-135

84) Raju RR, Goldblum JT, Hart WR. Pagetoid squamous cell carcinoma in situ {Pagetoid Bowen's disease} of the external genitalia Int J GynecolPathol 2003; 22:127-135

85) Fanning J Lambert HC, Hale TM, et al. Paget's disease of the vulva, prevalence associated vulvar adenocarcinoma, invasive Paget's disease, and recurrence after surgical excision. Am J ObstetGynecol 1999; 180:24-27

86) Wilkinson EJ, Brown HM. Vulvar Paget's disease of urothelial origin: a report of three cases and a proposed classification of vulvar Paget's disease. Hum Pathol 2002; 33:549-554

87) Zaino RJ, Nucci M, Kurman RJ. Diseases of the vagina in Blasuteins Pathology of the female genital tract, Kurman RJ, Ellenson LH, Ronnett BM (Eds), 6th Edition 2011, Springer pp 142-144

88) Hasumi K, Sakomoto G, Sugano H, et al. Primary malignant melanoma of the vagina: Study of four autopsy cases with ultrastructural findings. Cancer 1978; 42:2675-2686

89) Takagi M, Ishikawa G, Mori W. Primary malignant melanoma of the oral cavity in Japan with special reference to mucosal melanosis. Cancer 1974; 34:358-370

90) Etchepareborda FM, Sunn CC, Soliman PT, et al. Primary malignant melanoma of the vagina ObstetGynecol 2010; 116:1358-1365

91) Creasman WT, Phllips JL, Menck HR. The National Cancer Data Base Report on Cancer of the Vagina Cancer 1998; 83:1033-1040

92) Mousavi AS, Fakor F, Nazari Z, et al. Primary malignant melanoma of uterine cervix: case report and the review of the literature. J Low Genital Tract Dis.2006; 10:258-263

93) Yun NR, Park JW, Park JH, et al. Primary Malignant Melanoma of the Uterine Cervix: A Case Report. Korean J ObstetGynecol 2012; 55:343-347

94) Gupta R, Singh S, Mandal AK: Primary malignant melanoma of cervix: A
Case report Indian J Cancer 2005,42: 201-204.

95) Jones WH, Droegemuller W, Makowaski ELA. A primary melanocarcinoma of cervix.ObstetGynecol 1971; 111:959

Sarcoma Botryoides

96) Behtash N, Mousavi A, Tehranian A, et al Embryonal rhabdomyosarcoma of the uterine cervix; case report and review of the literature. GynecolOncol 2002; 91:452-455

97) Mousavi A, Akhavan S. Sarcoma botryoides (embryonal rhabdomyosarcoma) of the uterine cervix among sisters. J GynecolOncol 2010; 21:273-2754

98) Creasman WT, Phillips JL, Menck HR. The National Cancer Data Base Report on Cancer of the Vagina. Cancer 1998; 83:1033-1040

99) Fanghong R, Gupta M, McCluggage WG, et al. Embryonal Rhabdomyosarcoma (Botryoid Type) of the Uterine Corpus and Cervix in Adult Women. Report of a Case Series and Review of the Literature Am J SurgPathol 2013; 37:344-355

100) Copeland LJ, Sneige N, Stringer A, et al. Alveolar Rhabdomyosarcoma of the Female Genitalia. Cancer 1985; 56:849-855

Placental Site Trophoblastic Tumor (Trophoblastic Pseudotumor)

101) Kurman RJ, Scully RE, Norris NJ. Trophoblastic pseudotumor of the uterus: An exaggerated form of "syncitial endometritis" simulating a malignant tumor. Cancer1976; 7:1214-1226
102) Twiggs LB, Okagaki T, Phillips J, et al. Trophoblastic pseudotumor, evidence of malignant disease potential. GynecolOncol 1981; 12;238-248
103) Scully RE, Young RG: Trophoblastic pseudotumor. A reappraisal Am J SurgPathol 1981; 7:75-76
104) Goldstein DP. Gestational Trophoblastic Neoplasia in the 1990s The Yale Journal of Biology and Medicine 1991; 64:639-651
105) Behtash N, Ghaemmaghami F, Hasanzadeh M. Long term remission of metastatic placental site trophoblastic tumor (PSTT): Case report and review of literature World Journal of Surgical Oncology 2005; 3:34-37
106) Heyderman E, Gibbons AR, Rosen SW. Immunoperoxidase localization of human placental lactogen: a marker for the placental origin of the giant cells in 'syncitial endometritis' of pregnancy. J ClinPathol 1981; 34:303-307
107) Shih I-M, Kurman RJ (1998) Ki-67 labeling index in the differential diagnosis of exaggerated placental site, placental site trophoblastic tumor, and choriocarcinoma: a double immunohistochemical staining technique using Ki-67 and Mel-CAM antibodies. Hum Pathol 29:27–33
108) Young RH, Kurman RJ, Scully RE.Placental site nodules and plaques.A clinicopathologic analysis of 20 cases.Am J SurgPathol 1990; 14:1001–1009
109) Chang YL, Chang TC, Hsueh S, et al. Prognostic factors and treatment for placental site trophoblastic tumor: report of 3 cases and analysis of 88 cases. GynecolOncol 1999; 73:216–222

Surface Epithelial Tumors: Serous Borderline Tumor

110) Lee KR, Tavassoli FA, Prat J, Dietel M, Gersell DJ, Karseladze AI et al. Surface epithelial stromal tumors. In Tavassoli FA, Deville P (Ed.)Pathology and Genetics.Tumors of the Breast and Female Genital Organs. Edited by WHO Classification of Tumors, IARC Press, Lyon 2003,pp 117
111) Russell P Surface epithelial-stromal tumors of the ovary. IN: Kurman RJ (Ed) Blaustein'spathology of the female genital tract,1994, 4th Ed. Springer, New York, pp 493-532
112) McCluggage WG. Ovarian borderline tumours: a review with emphasis on controversial areas. Diagnostic Histopathol 2011;17:178-192
113) Bell DA, Scuhy RE. Ovarian serous borderline tumors with stromal microinvasion: a report of 21 cases Hum Pathol 1990 21:397-403
114) Bell DA, Weinstock MA, Scully RE. Peritoneal Implants of Ovarian Serous Borderline Tumors: Histopathologic Features and Prognosis. Cancer 1988; 62:2212-2222
115) Lettao MM. Micropapillary Pattern in Newly Diagnosed Borderline Tumors of the Ovary: What's in a Name? The Oncologist 2011; 16:133-135
116) Uzan C, Kane A, Rey A, et al. Prognosis and prognostic factors of the micropapillary pattern in patients treated for stage II and stage III Serous Borderline Tumors of the Ovary. The Oncologist 2011; 16:189-196
117) Seidman J, KurmanRJ.Subclassification of Serous Borderline Tumors of the Ovary Benign and Malignant types: A Clinicopathologic Study of 65 Advanced Stage Cases
118) Djordjevic B, Malpica A. Ovarian tumors of Low Malignant Potential with Nodal Low-grade Serous Carcinoma. Am J SurgPathol 2012; 00:00
119) Zinsser KR, Wheeler JE.Endosalpingiosis in the omentum: A study of autopsy and surgical material. Am J Surg Pathol 1982; 6:109-117
120) Kurman RJ, Vang R, Junge J, et al. Papillary Tubal Hyperplasia: The Putative Precursor of Ovarian Atypical Proliferative (Borderline) Serous Tumors, Noninvasive Implants and Endosalpingiosis
121) Siedman JD, Kurman RJ. Ovarian Serous Borderline Tumors: A critical Review of the Literature With Emphasis on Prognostic Indicators. Human Pathol 2000; 31:539-57

122) Eichorn JH, Bell DA, Young RH, et al. Ovarian serous borderline tumors with micropapillary and cribriform patterns: a study of 40 cases and comparison with 44 cases without these patterns. Am J SurgPathol 1999; 23:397-409

123) McCluggage WG. My approach to and thoughts on the typing of ovarian carcinomas. J ClinPathol 2008; 61:152-163

124) Kurman RJ, Shih IeM.Pathogenesis of ovarian cancer; lessons from morphology and molecular biology and their clinical implications.Int J GynecolPathol 2008; 27:15160

Mucinous tumors of ovary

125) Rodriguez IM, Prat J. Mucinous Tumors of the ovary: A clinicopathologic analysis of 75 borderline tumors (of intestinal type) and carcinomas. Am J SurgPathol 2002; 26:139-152

126) McCluggage WG. Ovarian borderline tumors: a review with emphasis on controversial areas. Diagnostic Histopathol 2011; 17:178-192

127) Riopel MA, Ronnett BM, Kurman RJ. Evaluation of Diagnostic Criteria and Behavior of Ovarian Intestinal-type Mucinous Tumors: Atypical Proliferative (Borderline) Tumors and Intraepithelial, Microinvasive, Invasive; and Metastatic carcinomas. Am J SurgPathol 1999; 23:617-635

128) Lee KR, Scully RE: A Clinicopathologic Study of 196 Borderline Tumors (of Intestinal Type) And Carcinomas, Including an Evaluation of 11 cases with 'Psuedomyxoma Peritonei. Am J SurgPathol 2000; 24:1447-1464

129) Guerrieri C, Hogberg T, Wingren S, et al. Mucinous and Borderline Malignant Tumors of the Ovary: A clinicopathologic and DNA Ploidy DNA Study of 92 cases.

130) Rodriguez IM, Irving JA, Prat J. Endocervical-like Mucinous Borderline Tumors of the Ovary: A clinicopathologic Analyses of 31 Cases. Am J SurgPathol 2004; 28:1311-1318

131) Young RH, Gilks B, Scully RE. Mucinous Tumors of the Appendix Associated with Mucinous Tumors of the Ovary and Pseudomyxoma Peritonei: A Clinicopathologic Analyses of 22 cases Supporting an Origin in the Appendix. Am J SurgPathol 1991; 15:415-429

132) Seidman J, Elsayed AM, Sobin LH et al. An association of Mucinous Tumors of Ovary and Appendix: A clinicopathologic study of 25 cases Am J SurgPathol 1993; 17:22-34

133) Carr NJ, McCarthy WF, Sobin LH. Epithelial non-carcinoid tumors and tumor like lesions of the appendix: a clinicopathologic study of 184 patients with multivariate analysis of prognostic factors. Cancer1995; 75:757-768

134) Ronnett BM, Shmookler BM, Diener-West M, et al Immunohistochemical evidence supporting the appendiceal origin pseudomyxomaperitonei in women. Int J GynecolPathol 1997; 16:1-9

135) Cuatrecasas M, Matias-Guiu X, Prat J. Synchronous mucinous tumors of the appendix and the ovary associated with psuedomyxomaperitonei: a clinicopathologic study of 6 cases with comparative analysis of c-Ki-rasmutations. Am J Surg Pathol 1996; 20:739-746

136) Ronnett BM, Zahn CM, Kurman RJ, et al. Disseminated peritoneal adenomucinosis and peritoneal mucinous carcinomatosis: a clinicopathologic analysis of 109 cases with emphasis on distinguishing pathologic features, site of origin, prognosis, and relationship to pseudomyxomaperitonei Am J SurgPathol 1995; 19:1390-1408

137) Ronnett BM, Yan H, Kurman RJ. Patients with pseudomyxomaperitonei associated with disseminated peritoneal adenomucinosis have a significantly more favorable prognosis than patients with peritoneal mucinous carcinomatosis. Cancer 2001; 92:85-91

Clear cell carcinoma of Ovary

138)Lee KR, Tavassoli FA, Prat J, Dietel M, Gersell DJ, Karseladze AI et al. Surface epithelial stromal tumors. In Tavassoli FA, Deville P (Ed.) Pathology and Genetics.Tumors of the Breast and Female Genital Organs IARC Press, Lyon 2003,pp 137-139

139) Carmen MG del, Birrer M, Schorge JO. Clear cell carcinoma of the ovary: A review of the literature. GynecolOncol 2012;126:481-90

140) Mao TL, Ayhan A, Ueda S, Lai H, Hayran M, Shih LeM et al Cystic and adenofibromatous clear cell carcinomas of the ovary: distinctive tumors that differ I their pathogenesis and behavior: a clinicopathologic analysis of 122 cases. Am J SurgPathol 2009;33:844-53

141) Offman SL, Longacre TA. Clear cell carcinoma of the female genital tract (not everything is as clear as it seems). AdvAnatPathol 2012;19:296-312

Gonadoblastoma

142) Scully RE. Gonadoblastoma: A Review of 74 cases. Cancer 1970; 25:1340-1356

143) Erhan Y, Toprak AS, Ozdemir N, et al. Gonadoblastoma and fertility. J ClinPathol; 1992:45:628—28

144) Hart WR, Burcans DM. Germ cell neoplasms arising in gonadoblastoma. Cancer 1979; 43:669-678

Metastatic Cancers in Ovary

145) Weber WB. Selected items from history of pathology.Friedrich Krukenberg and his tumor. Am J Pathol 1978; 93:792

146) Young RH, Hart WR. Metastases from cancers of the pancreas simulating primary mucinous tumor of the ovary Am J SurgPathol 1989; 13:748-756

147) Petru E, Pickel M, Heydarfadai Lahausen M, et al. Non-genital cancers metastatic to the ovary.GynecolOncol 1992; 44:83-86

148) Young RH, Scully RE. Mucinous ovarian tumors associated with mucinous adenocarcinoma of endocervix: a clinicopathologic analysis of 16 cases Int J GynecolPathol 1988; 7:99-111

149) Li W, Wang H, Wang J, et al. Ovarian metastases resection from extragenital primary sites: outcome and prognostic factor analysis of 147 patients BMC Cancer 2012; 12:278

150) Lee KR, Young RH. The distinction between primary and metastatic mucinous carcinomas of the ovary: Gross and histological findings in 50 cases Am J SurgPathol 2003; 27:281-292

151) Guerrieri C, Hogberg T, Wingren S, et al. Mucinous borderline and malignant tumors of the ovary: a clinicopathologic and DNA ploidy study of 92 cases Cancer 1994; 74:2329-2340

152) Scully RE, Lee KR. Mucinous tumors of the ovary: a clinicopathologic study of 196 borderline tumors (of intestinal type)and carcinomas including an evaluation of 11 cases of 'pseudomyxoma peritonei' Am J Surge Pathol 2000; 24:1447-1464

153) Riopel MA, Ronnet BM, Kurman RJ. Evaluation of diagnostic criteria and behavior of ovarian intestinal-type mucinous tumors: atypical proliferative (borderline) tumors and intraepithelial, microinvasive, and metastatic carcinoma Am J SurgPathol 1999; 23:617-635

154) Vang R, Gown AM, Barry TS, et al. Cytokeratins 7 and 20 in Primary and Secondary Mucinous tumors of the Ovary: Analysis of Coordinate Immunohistochemical Expression Profiles and Staining Distribution in 179 Cases Am J SurgPathol 2006; 30: 1130-1139

155) Berezowasky K, Stanstny JF, Kornstein MJ. Cytokeratins 7 and 20 and carcinoembryonic antigen in ovarian and colonic carcinoma. Mod Pathol 1996; 9:426-429

156) Dionigi A, Facco C, Tibiletti MG, et al. Ovarian metastases from colorectal carcinoma: clinicopathologic profile, Immunophenotype, and karyotype analysis. Am J ClinPathol 2000; 114: 111-122

157) LagendijkJH, Mullink H, Van Diest PJ, et al. Tracing the origin of adenocarcinomas with unknown primary using immunohistochemistry: differential diagnosis between colonic and ovarian carcinomas as primary sites. Hum pathol

158) Wauters CCAP, Smedst F, Gerritis LGM, et al. Keratin 7 and 20 as diagnostic markers of carcinoma metastatic to the ovary. Hum Pathol1995 ; 26:852-855

Aggressive angiomyxoma

159) Steeper TA, Rosai J. Aggressive Angiomyxoma of the female pelvis and perineum: Report of nine cases of a distinctive type of gynecologic soft-tissue neoplasm. Am J SurgPathol 1983; 7:463-475

160) Fetsch JF, Laskin WB, Lefkowitz M, et al. Aggressive Angiomyxoma: A clinicopathologic Study of 29 Female Patients. Cancer 1996; 78:79-80

161) Rawlinson NJ, West WW, Nelson M. Aggressive angiomyxoma with t(12:21) and HMGA2 Rearrangement: Report of a Case and Review of the Literature. Cancer Genet Cytogenet 2008; 181:119-124

162) Tsang WYW, Chan JKC, Lee KC, et al Aggressive Angiomyxoma: A Report of Four Cases Occurring in Men. Am J SurgPathol 1992; 16:1059-1065

163) Morag R, Fridman E, Mor Y. Aggressive Angiomyxoma of the Scrotum Mimicking Huge, Hydrocele: Case Report and Literature Review. Case Reports in Medicine 2009:Article 157624

164) Mathiesen A, Chandrakanth S, Yousef G, et al. Aggressive angiomyxoma of the pelvis: a case report J Can chir 2007; 50:228-229

165) McCluggage WG, Patterson A, Maxwell A Aggressive Angiomyxoma of pelvic parts exhibits oestrogen and progesterone receptor positivity. J ClinPathol 2000; 53:603-605

166) Kumar S, Agarwal N, Khanna R, et al. Aggressive angiomyxoma presenting with huge abdominal lump: A case report Cases Journal 2008 1:131-132

167) WHO Classification of Tumors, Pathology and Genetics, Tumors of Soft tissue and Bone (Ed) Fletcher CDM, Unni KK, Mertens F. IARC Press Lyon 2002 PP 189-90

PEComa

168) Folpe AL, Goodman ZD, Ishak K, et al Clear Myomelanocytic Tumor of the Falciform Ligament/Ligamentum Teres. A Novel Member of the Perivascular Epithelioid Clear cell Family of Tumors With a Predilection for Children and Young Adults Am J SurgPathol 2000; 24:1239-1246

169) Yang W, Li G, Zheng W-q. Multifocal PEComa (PECOmatosis) of the female genital tract and pelvis: a case report and review of the literature. Diagnostic pathology 2012; 7:23-27

170) Armah HB, Parwani AV. Malignant perivascular epithelioid cell tumor (PEComa) of the uterus with late renal and pulmonary metastases: a case report with review of the literature. Diagnostic Pathology 2007; 2:45-51

Molecular Pathogenesis of Ovarian carcinoma

171) Piek JM, van Diest PJ, Zweemer RP, et al. Dysplastic changes in prophylactically removed fallopian tubes of women predisposed to developing ovarian cancer. J Pathol 2001; 195:451-456

172) Lee Y, Miron A, Drapkin R, et al. A candidate precursor to serous carcinoma that originate in the distal fallopian tube J Pathol 2007; 211:26-35

173) Rabbab JT, Krasik E, Chen LM, et al. Multiple step sections to detect occult fallopian tube carcinoma in risk reducing salpingo-oophorectomies from women with BRCA mutations Implications for defining an optimal specimen dissection protocol. Am J SurgPathol 2009; 33:1878-1885

174) Shaw PA, Rouzbahman M, Pizer ES, et al. Candidate serous cancer precursors in fallopian tube epithelium of BRCA ½ mutation carriers. Mod Pathol 2009; 22L1133-1138

175) Finch A, Shaw PA, Rosen B, et al. Clinical and pathologic findings of prophylactic salpingo-oophorectomies in 159 BRCA 1 and BRCA 2 carriers. GynecolOncol 2006; 100:58-64

176) Carlson JW, Miron A, Jarboe EA, et al. Serous tubal intraepithelial carcinoma: its potential role in primary peritoneal serous carcinoma and serous cancer prevention. J ClinOncol 2008; 26:4160-4165

177) Alvarado-Cabrero I, Young RH, Vamvakas EC, et al. Carcinoma of the fallopian tube: A clinic0pathologic study of 105 cases with observations on staging and prognostic factors GynecolOncol 1999; 72:367-379

178) Mederios F, Muto MG, Lee Y, et al. The tubal fimbriae is the preferred site for early adenocarcinoma in women with familial ovarian cancer syndrome. Am J SurgPathol 2006; 30:230-236

179) Mehrad M, Ning G, ChenEY, et al. A pathologist's road map to benign, precancerous, and malignant intraepithelial proliferations in the fallopian tube AdvAnatPathol 2010; 17:293-302

180) Jarboe EA, Pizer ES, Miron A, et al Evidence for a latent precursor (p53 signature) that may precede serous endometrial intraepithelial carcinoma. Mod Pathol 2009; 22:345-350
